Passing the General Surgery Oral Board Exam

Marc A. Neff
Editor

Passing the General Surgery Oral Board Exam

Second Edition

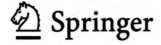

Editor
Marc A. Neff, M.D., F.A.C.S.
Minimally Invasive and Bariatric Surgeon
Cherry Hill, NJ, USA

ISBN 978-1-4614-7662-7   ISBN 978-1-4614-7663-4 (eBook)
DOI 10.1007/978-1-4614-7663-4
Springer New York Heidelberg Dordrecht London

Library of Congress Control Number: 2013944371

Printed on acid-free paper

Springer is part of Springer Science+Business Media (www.springer.com)

For Lauren, Jamie, Andrew, and Dylan

"Everyone falls down. Getting back up is how you learn how to walk."

—Walt Disney

Preface

"The American Board of Surgery regrets to inform you that you were not successful in the Certifying Examination given in Cleveland, OH, in October, 2002. It was the consensus of your examiners that your performance during the examination was not of the level required for certification by the Board."

That is the way the letter reads if you do not pass the Oral Boards from the American Board of Surgery. Three more paragraphs follow in that awful letter I read to myself the evening of November 2, 2002, less than 4 days since I had taken the Oral Boards. It was a cold fall night and all I could think of was, Why I didn't care more? Was it because a good friend had informed me earlier in the day that he had failed too? Was it that I just had such a bad gut instinct since I left the Board exam that I had been preparing myself the past few days for bad news? Who knows? After reading that letter, however, I did know one thing: The next time through, I would know everything there is to know about the field of general surgery so that there was no possible way I was going to fail a second time.

Out of that sentiment began the thoughts for this book. I could not sleep well that night after I opened the letter. As I thought about what I had done to prepare for the Boards, two review courses, flashcards, and a variety of review texts, I realized that the best help was a book entitled *Safe Answers for the Board*. This was really an excellent book that helped to clarify and crystallize a lot of what I learned in residency, and I recommend it to all potential Board examinees. I did realize after a search on the Internet, however, that there is no book that tells you what the wrong answers are, or what are the common curveballs that the examiners are likely to "throw" at you during the exam. My goal then became to put together a study guide to structure my review—one that not only reviewed the material necessary to pass the Oral Boards, but also to prepare an examinee for what actually happens at the Oral Board Exam.

I like to think that the underdog is always the better competitor in the final analysis. I knew that my failure did not mean I was less of a surgeon than those who passed. I knew it did not mean that I would not become a successful surgeon. I knew it did not mean that I was going to mismanage or kill my next hundred patients. I knew what it did mean—that I was going to "kick it" to those examiners at the Board of Surgery at the next exam. I will share with you a philosophy from my Philadelphia upbringing, being the home to many "underdogs" over the years: Who knows how to climb a ladder better: the person who climbed it first and never missed a step, or the person who climbs it, falls, and then climbs it again, paying close attention to ever rung on the ladder, every step of the way, because he knows what it feels like to fall and becomes determined never to fall again?

If I can offer a couple of suggestions for those of you preparing for this exam, they are the following:
1. Read a general surgery textbook cover to cover (any text, it really does not matter which text you choose)
2. Read lots of previous questions (you can get from any course or your colleagues)
3. Remember, self-induced anxiety is your biggest enemy

You passed the written exam, so you know the material. You just have to keep from freezing or getting tongue tied during the examination. Say what you would do if the question being asked was a real-life situation. This exam is more of a test of your thinking ability and confidence than a pure test of your knowledge—Can you process information and come up with a rational plan of action? You do this every day; you are not an "unsafe" surgeon. You just have to prove this to the examiners—in the archaic and overly subjective fashion called the Oral Board of Surgery Certification Exam—that you can verbally sum up 2 or more weeks of outpatient workup/inpatient care in about 7 minutes per question. Never make up answers or operations and do not waste time on history and physical examination if the examiner tells you, "That is all you need"—both are a sure way to fail. Remember, the exam starts right after the examiner shakes your hand.

Cherry Hill, NJ, USA   Marc A. Neff

Acknowledgements

It has been approximately 10 years since my achievement of board certification. Thinking back now, I am a little shocked at how innocent I was when I first conceived of this book. My world in 2003 was focused on simply getting four more initials after my name. That was a small accomplishment next to the trials of the past decade. I have survived contract negotiations, malpractice suits, remarkable patient successes, and terrible complications. I have fought with medical directors for insurance companies, built a successful surgical surgery program from the ground up, and been granted numerous awards, including top regional doctor several times over. I have a curriculum vitae now that is now pages long with publications/presentations, and I have inspired countless other medical students to pursue a career in surgery. I have even been hospitalized myself in an intensive care unit and seen what a hospitalized patient really experiences. All that has been on top of the more important "real-life" experiences, such as having children, buying and selling houses, and (sadly) watching my body change as I age.

Throughout it all, though, I remembered what it took to get this high on my mountain of achievements and never gave up climbing. That is the true measure of a surgeon, I'm convinced—the determination and tenacity to push yourself to the limits for others less fortunate every single day. In some ways, a surgeon is like a superhero. Superman could not control when the freight train went off the track, and he had to fly faster than a speeding bullet to save the passengers' lives. Well, neither can the surgeon control when the call comes from the answering service/resident for the emergent surgery for the free air. I understand the need for a fortress of solitude so much more now, and I have great empathy for Lois Lane.

My first thanks, as in the first edition, goes to my family. They are the ones who provide me with the support and stability that any surgeon needs to survive. Without them, I could not go to the hospital, work 14-hour days seven days a week, and expect to come home to any sort of stability in my life. They are the ones who never know how hard we surgeons struggle every day to get home by dinner time, or to be well groomed for family events, or to not forget someone's birthday. And yet, they still love us and have limitless patience for us while we are doing what we were born to do.

My second thanks belongs to my mentors for helping forge in me a foundation to help me survive and not succumb to the pressures inherent in being a surgeon. Through the past decade of true torture, they armored me and taught me how to fight the battle against surgical diseases and to adapt to the ever-changing medical paradigms. They could not foresee the future, but almost daily, I'm reminded of one or another lesson one of those "Jedi masters" taught me—a new fighting technique perhaps, or lightsaber defense—that can be reapplied to get me to survive the day's new challenges.

Lastly, I must thank the numerous contributors to this second edition. I am indebted to my partner, Dr. Linda Szczurek, for her contributions on the following sections: Choledochal Cyst, Choledocholithiasis, Gallstone Ileus, Acute and Chronic Pancreatitis, Pediatric Hernia, Neonatal Bowel Obstruction, Pyloric Stenosis, Tracheoesophageal Fistula, Nipple Discharge, Ductal Carcinoma In Situ, Inflammatory Breast Cancer, Invasive Ductal Carcinoma, Paget's Disease, Appendicitis, Ulcerative Colitis, and Cholecystitis. Dr. Anna Goldenberg Sandau and

Dr. Roy Sandau wrote very thorough reviews on Carcinoid, Cushing's Syndrome, Hyperthyroidism, Insulinoma, Pheochromocytoma, Primary Aldosteronism, Neck Mass, Hyperparathyroidism, and Thyroid Nodule. Dr. Christina Sanders provided excellent sections on Zenker's Diverticulum, Achalasia, Esophageal Cancer, Esophageal Perforation, Esophageal Varices, Gastroesophageal Reflux Disease, and Hiatal Hernia. Dr. Devin Flaherty provided wonderful reviews on Upper and Lower Gastrointestinal Bleeding, Rectal Cancer, and Colon Cancer. Dr. Nicole Harris provided thoracic expertise for Empyema and Lung Cancer. Dr. Jonathan Nguyen contributed to sections on Postoperative and Recent Myocardial Infarction, Pancreatic Cancer, and Pancreatic Pseudocyst. Dr. Thomas Cartolano provided insight into Rib Fracture, Extremity Compartment Syndrome, Genitourinary Trauma, and Pelvic Fracture. Drs. Leigh Ann Slater and Elliott Haut provided excellent sections on Duodenal Trauma, Liver Trauma, and Colon and Rectal Trauma. Drs. Luis Garcia and Elliott Haut provided thorough updates to the Splenic Trauma, Penetrating Neck Trauma, and Damage Control Surgery. Drs. Catherine Velopulos and Elliott Haut expertly reviewed Pulmonary Embolism. Drs. Farshad Farnejad and Elliott Haut updated the Thoracic Trauma section. Lastly, Dr. Brant Jones deserves special recognition for tackling the entire vascular section, including Abdominal Aortic Aneurysm (Rupture and Elective), Acute and Chronic Lower Extremity Ischemia, Carotid Stenosis, Deep Venous Thrombosis, and Venous Stasis Ulcer. To all my contributors, their tireless patience, energy, and determination have made this edition a success.

Cherry Hill, NJ, USA   Marc A. Neff

Contents

Contributors

Thomas Cartolano, D.O. General Surgery, University of Medicine and Dentistry of New Jersey, School of Osteopathic Medicine, Stratford, NJ, USA

Farshad Farnejad, M.D., M.P.H. Department of Surgery, Division of Acute Care Surgery, The Johns Hopkins University School of Medicine, Baltimore, MD, USA

Devin C. Flaherty, D.O., Ph.D. General Surgery, University of Medicine and Dentistry of New Jersey, School of Osteopathic Medicine, Stratford, NJ, USA

Luis J. Garcia, M.D. Department of Surgery, Division of Acute Care Surgery, The Johns Hopkins University School of Medicine, Baltimore, MD, USA

Nicole M. Harris, D.O., M.S. General Surgery, University of Medicine and Dentistry of New Jersey, School of Osteopathic Medicine, Stratford, NJ, USA

Elliott R. Haut, M.D., F.A.C.S. Department of Surgery, Division of Acute Care Surgery, The Johns Hopkins University School of Medicine, Baltimore, MD, USA

Brandt D. Jones, D.O. General Surgery, University of Medicine and Dentistry of New Jersey, School of Osteopathic Medicine, Stratford, NJ, USA

Marc A. Neff, M.D., F.A.C.S. Minimally Invasive and Bariatric Surgeon, Cherry Hill, NJ, USA

Jonathan Nguyen, D.O. General Surgery, University of Medicine & Dentistry of New Jersey, Stratford, NJ, USA

Anna Goldenberg Sandau, D.O. General Surgery, University of Medicine and Dentistry of New Jersey, School of Osteopathic Medicine, Stratford, NJ, USA

Roy L. Sandau, D.O. General Surgery, Kennedy University Hospital, Cherry Hill, NJ, USA

Christina Sanders, D.O. General Surgery, University of Medicine and Dentistry of New Jersey, School of Osteopathic Medicine, Stratford, NJ, USA

Leigh Ann Slater, M.D. Department of Surgery, Division of Acute Care Surgery, The Johns Hopkins University School of Medicine, Baltimore, MD, USA

Linda Szczurek, D.O., F.A.C.O.S. General Surgery Department, Kennedy Health System, Cherry Hill, NJ, USA

Catherine Garrison Velopulos, M.D. Department of Surgery, Division of Acute Care Surgery, The Johns Hopkins University School of Medicine, Baltimore, MD, USA

Organizational Theme

Marc A. Neff

Each chapter/topic will be organized as follows:

Concept—brief pathophysiologic discussion on the general surgery topic

Way Question May Be Asked—common scenario presentations and some variations on the theme

How to Answer—possible ways to answer the question based on a material reviewed, including multiple references, two review courses, and multiple experiences of actual examinees

Common Curveballs—possible ways the board examiners may challenge you. Be mindful of a change in scenario, when the examiner is satisfied with your answer but challenges you further by changing the results of your testing or your interventions. Remember, these are possible real-life situations, so just approach them as you would any patient in the hospital. Do not expect any question to end without at least one curveball on the oral boards.

Clean Kills—things not to miss, say, or fail to say; otherwise, you are likely coming back next year to try the examination again

Summary—most chapters now include an ending summary that embody some parting "words of wisdom" for the victim

---

Any Cancer

Concept

Make sure you understand the common nature of the spread of cancer (e.g., hematogenous—papillary/thyroid; peritoneal—ovarian; lymphatic—breast). All cancers need to be addressed with regard to the following:

Staging

Surgical treatment

(Neo)adjuvant therapies

M.A. Neff, M.D., F.A.C.S. (✉)
Minimally Invasive, 2201 Chapel Avenue West, Suite 100,
Cherry Hill, NJ 08002, USA
e-mail: mneffyhs@aol.com

Way Question May Be Asked?

Approximately half of the time, the diagnosis clearly will be cancer from the outset. For the other half of the questions, you will get the diagnosis unexpectedly after a long, exhaustive workup.

How to Answer?

As with everything else, be methodical.

For *history,* do not leave out important systemic symptoms such as change in bowel habits, dysphagia, weight loss, anorexia, jaundice, last mammogram, and family history of malignancies.

For *physical examination,* do not leave out important information such as abdominal masses, examination of important lymphatic basins, or complete skin examination for a patient with melanoma

Make sure you do everything you can for the patient in the preoperative workup:

1. Determine a diagnosis (e.g., fine needle aspiration [FNA], ultrasound, mammogram for breast cancer)
2. Determine appropriate staging (but do not go overboard with ordering tests!)
   (a) Liver function tests and chest x-ray (CXR) for breast cancer
   (b) Pulmonary function tests and computed tomography (CT) scan from chest to adrenals for lung cancer, with or without mediastinoscopy
   (c) CT scan of the abdomen/pelvis, angiography, tumor markers, and endoscopic retrograde cholangiopancreatography (ERCP) for pancreatic cancer
3. Determine if lesion is resectable or if patient needs preoperative chemotherapy/radiotherapy
   (a) Patients with rectal cancer of stage II or greater need preoperative radiotherapy
   (b) Patients with inflammatory breast cancer need preoperative chemotherapy

M.A. Neff (ed.), *Passing the General Surgery Oral Board Exam,*
DOI 10.1007/978-1-4614-7663-4_1, © Springer Science+Business Media New York 2014

If you do not have a diagnosis yet in the operating room (as in the case of a pancreatic mass), you must do frozen section.

A frozen section also is appropriate after resection to check margins in gastric, esophageal, and lung cancer.

Examine lymph node basins when appropriate.

Frozen sections of sentinel lymph nodes (SLNs) are controversial for cancers other than melanoma and breast. There is not necessarily a right answer, but know your answer and stick to it!

Be able to describe common lymph node dissections.

Do not forget to ask for a pathology report—size, margins, lymph nodes, tumor type, and nuclear grade (receptor status for breast cancer).

Do not forget to discuss postoperative chemotherapy/radiotherapy management.

Common Curveballs

Cancer diagnosis that is unable to be determined preoperatively (common with pancreatic/cholangiocarcinoma)

Margins positive in gastric/breast cancer

Mediastinoscopy positive

Postoperative 1 year with local recurrence or rising tumor markers in first year of postoperative follow-up

Postoperative 1 year with metastatic lesion (resect in sarcoma if primary site is controlled and in melanoma if there is single-organ metastasis)

Postoperative discussion of chemotherapy/radiotherapy regimen

"Scenario switch" in which you were working up one diagnosis and find a malignancy

(e.g., Bloody nipple discharge after resection, path reveals small focus ductal carcinoma)

Patient has synchronous tumor in colon cancer

Patient has postoperative leak after gastrointestinal (GI) resection

Patient with advanced breast cancer wants to preserve her breast

Patient has positive SLN on permanent/frozen section

Patient has nondiagnostic FNA or percutaneous biopsy

Describe your technique for performing SLN biopsies

Clean Kills

Failure to check old CXR if lung cancer is suspected

Failure to check old mammogram or order mammogram for breast cancer

Failure to complete lymph node dissection for positive SLN (do not get into discussion about most recent National Surgical Adjuvant Breast and Bowel Project trials that randomize patients to not have complete axillary lymph node dissection for positive SLN in breast cancer)

Failure to know chemo/radiotherapy regimen after resection for breast cancer

Failure to check margins after GI resection

Aggressive resection of metastatic lesions in breast cancer

Failure to do FNA on palpable thyroid nodule/breast lesion

Failure to get preoperative lymphoscintigraphy if performing SLN for trunk melanoma (can go to at least four different lymph node basins)

Failure to use preoperative radiotherapy in rectal cancer stage II or greater

Failure to evaluate adrenal glands in evaluation of lung cancer

Failure to preoperatively determine resectability for a patient with pancreatic neoplasm

Failure to examine lymph node basins during preoperative history and physical examination

Failure to ask about prior history of malignancy during preoperative history and physical examination

Breast

Linda Szczurek

Nipple Discharge

Concept

Nipple discharge can be from benign or malignant causes. Benign discharge typically is nonspontaneous, bilateral, clear or milky, and from multiple ducts. Bloody discharge typically is caused by an intraductal papilloma (45 %), duct ectasia (35 %), or infection (~5 %), but it may be cancer (~5 %; this is a common curveball).

Way Question May Be Asked?

"A 45-year-old woman presents to your office with the complaint of unilateral bloody nipple discharge for the past one month."

When given just the complaint of nipple discharge, you should work through type, spontaneity, laterality, and recent medications that have been started. The question may also be concerning nipple discharge in a young woman.

How to Answer?

Full history
    Whether discharge occurs when stimulated or spontaneous (spontaneous is worrisome)
    Risk factors for malignancy
    Trauma
    Fluid characteristics (clear, milky, serous, bloody)
    Bilateral or unilateral

L. Szczurek, D.O., F.A.C.O.S. (✉)
General Surgery Department, Kennedy Health System,
2201 Chapel Avenue West, Suite 100, Cherry Hill, NJ 08002, USA
e-mail: lszczurek@hotmail.com

Discharge from one duct or multiple ducts
Trauma
Thyroid disorder
Recent new medications
Any other symptoms such as pain, swelling, or masses
Full physical examination
    Examination of both breasts in upright and supine positions
    Examination of lymph node basins
    Try to determine a responsible quadrant/responsible ducts
    The color and nature of the fluid
    The number of ducts producing fluid (multiple is usually benign, whereas single has higher risk of cancer)
Diagnostic tests
    Mammogram (mandatory)
    Ultrasound (subareolar area images poorly on mammogram)
    Hemoccult test
    Cytology (rarely helpful, and negative result does not exclude malignancy)
    Ductogram (painful and rarely helpful)
    Magnetic resonance imaging (MRI; rarely helpful for papilloma, but may detect other lesions)
For bloody discharge, you are in one of several situations:

1. Negative mammogram, negative physical examination for mass, and negative responsible quadrant:
Have patient follow-up in several weeks and check for responsible quadrant on breast self-examination. Then, on follow-up, consider the following situations:
   (a) Negative mammogram, positive physical examination for mass, and negative responsible quadrant:
   Total subareolar ductal system resection
   (b) Negative mammogram, positive physical examination for mass, and positive responsible quadrant:
   Subareolar wedge resection of ductal system for that quadrant
   (c) Positive mammogram, positive physical examination for mass, and positive responsible quadrant:
   Excisional biopsy of mass and subareolar wedge resection

2. Negative mammogram, positive physical examination, for mass, and positive responsible quadrant:
   Subareolar wedge resection of the ductal system draining that quadrant
3. Positive mammogram, positive physical examination for mass, and positive responsible quadrant:
   Excisional biopsy or core-needle biopsy of mass on mammogram and subareolar wedge resection

Surgical Procedure

Circumareolar incision (some surgeons make the incision at the nipple/areola border)

Elevate areola

Dissect ducts leading to areola

Identify abnormal duct by dilatation, stent, dye, or mass (if you can identify single duct, otherwise subareolar wedge resection of the ductal system draining that quadrant)

Tie off distal duct or it will still drain out of nipple postoperatively (your seroma!)

Common Curveballs

The pathology is not a benign intraductal papilloma but rather a type of breast cancer, which may range from lobular carcinoma in situ and ductal carcinoma in situ (DCIS) to invasive cancer. Do not forget about checking lymph nodes and adjuvant therapy!

The nipple discharge persists after a subareolar wedge resection. Early recurrence may be drainage of a seroma; the other possibility is that not all of the duct was excised.

There is not be a responsible quadrant.

There is a mass in the same breast, different quadrant, or in the opposite breast. Always treat the cancer first.

Discharge is not bloody but there are persistent atypical cells on slide cytology. (Now what do you do?)

Patient is pregnant (can have bloody nipple discharge during third trimester).

Patient is a teenager.

Clean Kills

Performing surgery for nonspontaneous, bilateral, clear/milky discharge

Failing to check the same breast for palpable masses or examine the other breast

Failing to establish risk factors for malignancy

Failing to check nodal status if pathology returns malignancy

Failing to order a mammogram/ultrasound

Discussing ductoscopy

Performing mastectomy for bloody nipple discharge

Not being able to shift into discussion of malignancy if pathology does not reveal expected papilloma but rather an invasive carcinoma

Trusting slide cytology/hemoccult tests and not performing surgery on patient with suspicious nipple discharge

Wasting time working up a prolactinoma

Summary

When evaluating a any patient with a breast complaint, a thorough history is key. The most important factors are the type of drainage and whether or not the discharge is spontaneous. Mammogram, ultrasound, cytology, and ductography may be helpful but the definitive diagnosis is made via excision of the involved duct. It is very important to rule out a concurrent malignancy.

Ductal Carcinoma In Situ

Concept

DCIS is a pre-malignant lesion with various subtypes. A patient has about a 33 % chance of developing invasive ductal carcinoma in their lifetime. Several key features from a pathologic standpoint include size of tumor, unifocal or multifocal, nuclear grade, necrosis, and level of differentiation.

Way Question May Be Asked?

"A 51-year-old woman presents to your office with an abnormal mammogram. A cluster of five microcalcifications were present in the upper outer quadrant of the left breast. She underwent a core-needle biopsy that revealed DCIS. What would you do?"

You may be given DCIS in a number of different ways, such as by a mammogram showing asymmetric density, nodule, and speculated lesion, but most commonly from clustered or branching heterogenous microcalcifications.

How to Answer?

For history, establish risk factors for breast cancer (menarche, breast-feeding, family history of breast/ovarian/prostate cancer, number of children, previous breast cancer, menopause, history of birth control pills or hormone replacement therapy, history of radiation, age at first pregnancy)

For physical examination, be sure to check both breasts.

Assess symmetry, dimpling, and erythema.

Try to palpate for any masses.

Examine for cervical/axillary/supraclavicular adenopathy.

Consider the need to order bilateral mammograms and compare to previous.

Ultrasound is useful for palpable masses to determine if they are cystic or solid.

MRI is not used for screening purposes.

Any suspicious microcalcifications (clustered, branching, heterogeneous) need to be biopsied (stereotactic core needle or needle localization/excisional biopsy).

After biopsy has identified the lesion as DCIS, the patient still needs that area to be excised with adequate (>2–5 mm) free margins. If you do not get this after your needle localization, you will need to re-excise until you begin to distort the breast or you get free margins.

If DCIS is diffuse—multifocal (scattered in one quadrant) or other quadrants (multicentric)—the patient will need total mastectomy.

If the tumor is high grade, has comedo necrosis, or is large/multifocal, a total mastectomy is appropriate (no axillary lymph node dissection [ALND] is necessary here unless the final path reveals invasive carcinoma). Be sure to offer immediate reconstruction as an option.

The patient will need postoperative radiotherapy (unless she had mastectomy or has a low-grade, small tumor with > 1 cm margin) to the breast and should be placed on 5 years of tamoxifen (unless contraindicated, such as in endometrial cancer or history of deep venous thrombosis).

Common Curveballs

There is a palpable mass (separate from mammographic finding).

There is more than one mammographically detected lesion.

There is a lesion in the opposite breast.

The patient has a recurrence after mastectomy to chest wall or incision site (scenario switch).

The patient has invasive carcinoma (scenario switch).

On pathology, the resection margin is positive or less than 1 mm.

The patient is pregnant.

Stereotactic core cannot be performed (too superficial, too deep, or the patient cannot lay prone on stereotactic table).

Lobular carcinoma in situ is shown on final pathology (maybe even at margins).

Clean Kills

Forgetting to examine both breasts

Forgetting to order bilateral mammograms

Forgetting postoperative chemotherapy/radiotherapy treatment when appropriate

Forgetting ALND if invasive cancer is identified

Not knowing indications for mastectomy in a patient with DCIS

Performing ALND for DCIS

Talking about sentinel lymph node biopsy for comedo DCIS (only in research protocols currently)

Talking about use of chemotherapy or the new medication you read about in a journal last week in an experimental trial for your patient with DCIS

Summary

A full history to establish the patient's risk factors for breast cancer and a complete examination of both breasts and the lymph node basins are very important. For DCIS, bilateral mammogram and other imaging techniques will be key. Suspicious lesions on mammogram need to be biopsied and subsequently excised with greater than 2–5 mm margins. Patients are then treated with radiation and hormone therapy.

Inflammatory Breast Cancer

Concept

Inflammatory breast cancer has poor prognosis regardless of the type of therapy offered. You do want to try to provide local control. You need to look for tumor cells in subdermal lymphatics (lymphovascular invasion) and treat aggressively. Differential diagnosis includes mastitis, abscess, and Mondor's disease.

Way Question May Be Asked?

"A 58-year-old woman presents to your office complaining of a breast infection. Examination reveals an erythematous, edematous right breast. What do you want to do?" The question may also include a failed course of antibiotics, a history of trauma, or recent breastfeeding/nursing to try to lead you astray.

How to Answer?

History
    Risk factors
        Menarche
        Breast-feeding
        Family history of breast cancer
        Number of children

Previous breast cancer

Menopause

History of birth control pills or hormone replacement therapy

History of radiation

Age at first pregnancy

Important questions include the following:

History of trauma

Nursing

Time course

Breast self-examinations (palpable masses before inflammation?)

Physical examination

Examine both breasts (peau d'orange)

Examine lymph node basins (cervical/axillary)

Palpable cord (Mondor's disease)

Diagnostic tests (as in all breast questions!)

Mammogram (bilateral)

Ultrasound (if mass)

MRI (usually for palpable lesion not seen on mammogram or ultrasound)

Differential diagnosis

Mastitis

Breast abscess

Superficial thrombophlebitis (palpable cord)

Inflammatory breast cancer

Surgical Treatment

1. It is acceptable to try a short course of antibiotics (1 week)
2. If symptoms fail to resolve or there is a strong suspicion for cancer, get an incisional biopsy (including skin) through the reddened area and include adjacent normal skin. Some clinicians recommend fine needle aspiration (FNA) because clinical grounds confirm the stage of disease and you just want a diagnosis of cancer to start chemotherapy. However, you will get more information from a core needle or incisional biopsy, including ER/PR receptor status.
3. If pathology confirms inflammatory breast cancer (tumor in subdermal lymphatics), proceed with metastatic workup as follows:
   (a) Chest x-ray
   (b) Computed tomography scan of the head, abdomen, and pelvis (look for metastases)
   (c) Bone scan
   (d) With or without positron emission tomography (PET) scan
4. Three cycles of chemotherapy (usually multi-agent)
5. Algorithm
   (a) If the patient has a complete response, perform a modified radical mastectomy to augment local control,

followed by eight cycles of chemotherapy, chest wall radiation, and tamoxifen if ER/PR positive.
   (b) If the patient has no response, then perform chest wall radiation and modified radical mastectomy.
6. If the tumor is already eroding through skin, you can give upfront radiotherapy to shrink tumor (also works if grossly eroding through skin and infected).

Common Curveballs

Erosion through skin during treatment

Patient does not have response to chemotherapy

Patient is pregnant

Patient somewhat responds during antibiotic treatment

Patient has mass or abnormal mammogram for opposite breast

Patient develops deep vein thrombosis during chemotherapy (scenario switch)

Patient pushes to save her breast or have immediate reconstruction (no!)

FNA is positive but you cannot get any receptor information (need to do core or incisional biopsy)

Clean Kills

Performing FNA instead of incisional biopsy (need receptor status)

Not recognizing inflammatory breast cancer as a T4 lesion

Not performing biopsy but proceeding straight to chemotherapy

Not performing mastectomy at end of neoadjuvant therapy (even if complete clinical resolution)

Not treating first with chemotherapy but proceeding straight with mastectomy

Talking about MRI (PET scan is only appropriate here for complete staging purposes)

Trying breast conservation/breast reconstruction

Summary

Unlike ductal and lobular carcinoma of the breast, inflammatory breast cancer has a poor prognosis and is diagnosed via lymphovascular invasion on biopsy. A thorough history should be obtained. On examination, the breast is usually erythematous and edematous with possible peau d'orange. Standard imaging with bilateral mammogram should be obtained, followed by biopsy. If the biopsy is positive, a metastatic workup should be completed. Again, although the prognosis is poor, the treatment is normally a combination of mastectomy, chemotherapy, radiation, and hormone therapy, depending on receptor status.

Invasive Ductal Carcinoma

Concept

Invasive ductal carcinoma is a malignancy that needs complete staging workup and then adjuvant treatment. Most women are candidates for breast conservation therapy (BCT), but you need to know the contraindications to BCT.

Way Question May Be Asked?

"A 45-year-old woman presents to your office with a palpable mass in the upper outer quadrant of the right breast. What would you do?"

You will likely be presented with a patient who has either a palpable abnormality, a locally advanced lesion, or a suspicious mammographic abnormality. Just be systematic and do what you would normally do in your practice.

How to Answer?

History
    Risk factors for breast cancer Menarche
        Breast-feeding
        Family history of breast cancer
        Number of children
        Previous breast cancer
        Menopause
        History of birth control pills or hormone replacement therapy
        History of radiation
        Age at first pregnancy
        Symptoms: bone pain, weight loss
        Change in breast appearance
    For the physical examination, assess symmetry, dimpling, erythema, and edema.
    Try to palpate any mass (hard/soft, well circumscribed, mobile/fixed, tender).
    Be sure to check both breasts!
    Examine for cervical/axillary adenopathy.
    Examine liver.
How to Answer
    You need to order bilateral mammograms and compare to any previous mammograms.
    Ultrasound is useful for palpable masses to determine if cystic or solid (especially in premenopausal breasts and may show characteristics of malignancy).
    The role of MRI is still controversial: 13–15 % of patients with one tumor are found to have another mass on MRI.
    FNA can be done in the office setting for any palpable lesion.

Core-needle biopsy can be done in the office or under stereotactic/ultrasound guidance. It is better than FNA because it provides information on invasion, hormone receptor status, tumor grade, and sometimes lymphovascular invasion.
Excisional biopsy should be performed on the following:
Solid mass
Cyst with bloody content
Cyst that recurs more than twice
    If FNA reveals malignancy, then you can plan full cancer staging in one trip to the operating room.
Contraindications for breast conservation therapy
    Tumor $\geq$ 5 cm
    Large tumor-to-breast ratio (cosmetic outcome)
    Two or more primary tumors in separate quadrants (multifocal)
    Previous breast irradiation
    Collagen vascular disease (scleroderma or lupus cannot get radiotherapy)
    Diffuse suspicious or indeterminate calcifications
    Subareolar tumor
    First and second trimester of pregnancy

Surgical Options

1. Lumpectomy (with clear margins), ALND, and postoperative radiotherapy
2. Modified radical mastectomy (combines total mastectomy and ALND)

ALND includes level 1 and 2 (lateral to and behind the pectoralis minor muscle) and should be done in all patients.
Sentinel lymph node biopsy is now an accepted technique. However, if frozen section or final pathology is positive, you would proceed to complete ALND.
Adjuvant chemotherapy treatment (combination of docetaxel/doxyrubicin/cyclophosphamide) is appropriate for the following patients:

1. All premenopausal women with invasive breast cancer > 1 cm in size
2. All postmenopausal women with positive lymph nodes
3. Postmenopausal women with T2 or greater lesions (>2 cm in size)

Adjuvant hormonal treatment is appropriate for the following patients:

1. All premenopausal women with invasive breast cancer >1 cm in size
2. All postmenopausal women (unless contraindicated)

Adjuvant radiotherapy decreases local recurrence but offers no difference in overall survival.

1. Use 5,000 rad in divided doses to the chest wall in all patients who underwent BCT. You cannot

administer during pregnancy, but you can usually delay until after pregnancy.

2. When more than four lymph nodes are involved with the tumor, radiotherapy to the axilla reduces local recurrence.

For pathology results, you need to know tumor characteristics: nuclear grade, vascular invasion, tumor size, ER/PR receptors, S-phase fraction, Her-2 Ne.

Staging

T1: less than or equal to 2 cm

T2: greater than 2 cm but less than or equal to 5 cm

T3: greater than 5 cm

T4: any size extending to the chest wall or skin

N1: movable same side axillary lymph nodes

N2: fixed same side axillary lymph nodes

N3: same side infraclavicular or inferior mammary and axillary same side or same side supraclavicular lymph nodes

M0: no distant metastasis

M1: distant metastasis

Galen Model for Chemotherapy

Low risk: node negative, grade 1 tumor, <2 cm, no lymphovascular invasion, ER+ and/or PR+, Her2Neu negative, for which endocrine therapy is indicated

Intermediate: node negative, does not fit in low risk, ER+ and/or PR+, Her2Neu negative, for which endocrine therapy is the primary treatment but you can consider chemotherapy

High risk: node positive, for which the patient should receive chemotherapy and endocrine therapy; Her2Neu-positive patients should get trastuzumab

Common Curveballs

There is a separate mammographic finding.

There is a palpable lesion not seen on mammogram.

There is a lesion in the opposite breast.

The patient has a recurrence after your surgical treatment.

Pulmonary/liver metastatectomy is not performed

Margins are positive for cancer or DCIS (or less than 1 mm)

Sentinel node biopsy does not work or is the only positive lymph node

Patient is pregnant (no radiotherapy, sentinel lymph node biopsy, or antimetabolite-based chemotherapy);

can give AC (adriomycin cytoxan) after late first trimester (only antimetabolite methotrexate unsafe during pregnancy);

no radiotherapy until the patient delivers (needs 24 weeks chemotherapy so ok unless <14 weeks pregnant);

no Tamoxifen or bone scan

Patient has contraindication to BCT

Patient has contraindication to adriamycin (poor ejection fraction)

Patient initially presents with nipple discharge

Patient has clinically positive axillary nodes

Patient has very strong family history (discussion of BRCA1, 2)

Cancer presents in a cyst that had bloody fluid on FNA

Patient has retroarealor cancer (will you perform mastectomy?)

Postmenopausal patient has T1 lesion, lymph nodes are negative but receptors are unfavorable (will you give chemotherapy?)

Postmenopausal patient has T2 lesion and receptors are favorable (will you give chemotherapy and/or hormonal therapy?)

Clean Kills

Forgetting to examine both breasts

Forgetting to order bilateral mammograms

Not asking about receptors on pathology

Forgetting postoperative chemo/radiotherapy treatment when appropriate

Forgetting ALND if invasive cancer is identified

Going into lengthy discussion about sentinel lymph node biopsy when you do not do these routinely in your practice

Performing therapeutic abortion for breast cancer in the pregnant patient

Not knowing contraindications to BCT

Not knowing who gets adjuvant treatment and with what chemotherapy/hormonal agents

Not recognizing stage IIIB breast cancer; sign include chest wall invasion, inflammatory breast cancer and skin ulceration.

Summary

The treatment of breast cancer requires a complete history; physical examination that includes bilateral breasts, lymph node basins, and liver; bilateral mammogram; and biopsy of the lesion. Core needle biopsy yields more information than FNA. In the appropriate patients, studies have shown that breast conservation therapy and mastectomy have equal survival. There are several contraindications to breast conservation therapy. The definitive combination of surgical and oncological treatment ultimately depends on the size and location of the mass/masses as well as the lymph node status.

Paget's Disease

Concept

These malignant cells have migrated from underlying DCIS or invasive cancer. Paget's cells are identified in the epidermis. They may regress with topical steroids, so do not prescribe them! Bilateral eczematous changes to the nipple areolar complex (NAC) are likely benign. Approximately 50 % of patients with Paget's disease will have an associated invasive cancer or DCIS. Only 10 % of patients will have disease confined to the nipple.

Way Question May Be Asked?

"A 43-year-old woman presents to your office with a 4-week history of itching to her left nipple. Examination reveals a reddened eczematous left nipple-areola complex (NAC) and a 1.5 cm mass in the upper outer quadrant approximately 4 cm from the NAC margin. What would you do?" There may or may not be an associated mass, but you should always perform a physical examination and mammogram/ultrasound.

How to Answer?

History
    Risk factors for breast cancer
        Menarche
        Breast-feeding
        Family history of breast cancer
        Number children
        Previous breast cancer
        Menopause
        History of birth control pills or hormone replacement therapy
        History of radiation
        Age at first pregnancy
Physical examination
    Try to palpate a mass
    Check both breasts!
    Examine for cervical/axillary adenopathy
How to Answer
    You need to order bilateral mammograms.
    A couple of situations are possible:
      1. No palpable mass and no lesions on mammography: Perform a wedge resection of NAC and check pathology. If Paget's cells are identified, you should proceed to simple mastectomy. If there is cancer in the mastectomy specimen, do not forget the ALND.

      2. Palpable mass or lesion on mammogram: Perform a wedge resection of NAC and excisional biopsy of mass. If Paget's cells are identified and mass is invasive cancer, then perform a modified radical mastectomy.

      3. Palpable mass or lesion on mammogram: Perform a wedge resection of NAC and excisional biopsy of mass. If Paget's cells are identified and mass is DCIS, then perform a simple mastectomy.

Do not forget radiation/chemotherapy/hormonal therapy when appropriate for DCIS or underlying invasive cancer.

Common Curveballs

There is a palpable mass.
There is a mammographically detected lesion.
There is a lesion in the opposite breast.
The patient has a recurrence after mastectomy to chest wall or incision site (scenario switch).

Clean Kills

Forgetting to order mammograms
Forgetting postoperative chemotherapy/radiotherapy treatment when appropriate
Forgetting ALND if invasive cancer is identified
Forgetting to obtain usual history/physical examination (establish risk factors, check masses in both breasts)
Forgetting to examine both breasts/axillae
Treating nipple with steroids (Paget's can remit on steroids)

Summary

Paget's disease presents as a eczematous lesion of the nipple areolar complex. Although it may appear to be focal, Paget's often extends past the NAC and is frequently associated with DCIS or invasive cancer. The same routine should be followed as with all other breast cancers, including a thorough history, physical examination, and mammogram. If Paget's cells are identified on the wedge resection of the NAC, the definitive treatment is simple mastectomy.

Colon and Small Bowel

Linda Szczurek, Devin C. Flaherty, and Marc A. Neff

Acute Bowel Ischemia

Concept

The pathogenesis of acute bowel ischemia includes multiple etiologies that can generally be broken down into occlusive and nonocclusive types. The differential diagnosis (DDx) for a patient with suspected colonic ischemia should also include other colonic disorders such as ulcerative colitis, infectious colitis, and pseudomembranous colitis. A breakdown of important types of occlusive and nonocclusive ischemia follows:

Occlusive	Nonocclusive
Embolism	Hypovolemia
Thrombosis	Cardiac failure/cardiogenic shock
Vascular compression	Hypotension
Abdominal aortic aneurysm repair	

Watershed areas vulnerable to low flow states in the colon include Griffith's point (splenic flexure) and Sudeck's point (rectosigmoid) for nonocclusive ischemia.

L. Szczurek, D.O., F.A.C.O.S. (✉)
General Surgery Department, Kennedy Health System,
2201 Chapel Avenue West, Suite 100, Cherry Hill, NJ 08002, USA
e-mail: lszczurek@hotmail.com

D.C. Flaherty, D.O., Ph.D.
General Surgery, University of Medicine and Dentistry of New Jersey, School of Osteopathic Medicine, Stratford, NJ, USA
e-mail: flaherde@umdnj.edu

M.A. Neff, M.D., F.A.C.S.
Minimally Invasive and Bariatric Surgeon,
2201 Chapel Avenue West, Suite 100, Cherry Hill, NJ 08002, USA
e-mail: mneffyhs@aol.com

Way Question May Be Asked?

"You are called to see a 54-year-old man on postoperative day 2 after an uncomplicated AAA repair with a massive bloody bowel movement. What do you want to do?"

Situation could also be after recent open heart surgery, recent myocardial infarction (MI), or a more chronic form with postprandial pain for several months with associated weight loss. Remember that pain out of proportion to physical examination is a classic sign for acute bowel ischemia. Try to separate generalized intestinal ischemia from colonic ischemia and occlusive from low flow states.

How to Answer?

History
    Inquire about the following risk factors:
    Valvular disease, coronary artery disease, hypercoagulable state, cardiac arrhythmias
    Classic: abrupt onset abdominal pain, diarrhea, hematochezia
    Recent surgery (AAA, bypass)
    Recent MI (embolus)
    Classic triad of fever, abdominal pain, and heme-positive stools
    Abrupt onset of pain, diarrhea, hematochezia
Physical examination
    "Toxic" appearance, shock, acidosis, leukocytosis
    Pain out of proportion to physical examination
    Peritonitis
    Heme-positive stools
    Gross blood (usually late finding)
    Irregular heart rate (atrial fibrillation)
Diagnostic tests
    Full laboratory tests (amylase and lactate also helpful)—acidosis is a late finding

M.A. Neff (ed.), *Passing the General Surgery Oral Board Exam*,
DOI 10.1007/978-1-4614-7663-4_3, © Springer Science+Business Media New York 2014

Electrocardiogram (EKG, to rule out atrial fibrillation)

Abdominal x-ray (AXR): free air, pneumatosisintestinalis, portal vein air

Computed tomography (CT) scan: "thumb printing," bowel wall thickening, pneumatosis, portal vein air

Colonoscopy: mucosal edema, submucosal hemorrhage, mucosal ulceration, bluish-black discoloration, areas of black nonviable mucosa, possible skip areas (keep air insufflation to a minimum, may prep with gentle tap water enema)

Arteriography (to evaluate small bowel):

Could see superior mesenteric artery (SMA) embolus

Could see SMA thrombosis

Could see normal proximal vessels but then distal spasm

Surgical Treatment

1. Decide if this is an acute mesenteric occlusion or colonic ischemia.
2. Initial steps include the following:

   Volume support (may need swan-ganz catheter (SGC)), intensive care unit, oxygen, bowel rest, nasogastric tube (NGT), Foley catheter

   Serial laboratory work/examinaions

   Antibiotics when remarkable endoscopic findings or toxemia
3. If colonic ischemia improves, then perform a colonoscopy 6–8 weeks later to evaluate for resolution/sequelae (stricture). Approximately 5 % of patients have recurrent episodes.
4. If patient becomes toxic or shows peritoneal signs, resuscitate patient and prepare for operating room (OR).

   In the OR, consider the following:

   Control contamination

   Palpation of celiac, SMA, inferior mesenteric artery (IMA) pulses

   Pattern of ischemia may suggest etiology (complete vs. patchy)

   Hand-held Doppler, fluorescein injection/Wood's lamp, warm packs

   Left colon involvement: resection with colostomy plus mucous fistula or Hartmann's pouch

   Right colon involvement: resection with ileostomy and mucous fistula

   Perform a second-look laparotomy if there is any question of viability

   Facts on aortic surgery include the following:

   Ischemia complicates 1–2 % of elective cases

   50 % mortality rate

   Early colonoscopy

   Reimplantation of IMA should be performed when there is severe SMA diagnosis, enlarged IMA, loss of Doppler

in sigmoid mesentery, history of prior colon resection, poor IMA back bleeding (stump pressure<40 mmHg)

If you need to take the patient back to the OR, perform end colostomy and Hartman pouch.

5. For small bowel ischemia, if the patient is toxic or angiogram is positive (angiogram is helpful in situations of suspected small bowel ischemia, not for ischemic colitis), proceed to OR as follows:

   Prepare access to greater saphenous vein in thigh

   Expose SMA

   (a) SMA embolus (proximal braches of SMA are spared)

   Seen 3–8 cm from SMA origin (spares first portion of jejunum only)

   Perform embolectomy through transverse arteriotomy

   Administer postoperative heparin

   Perform "second-look" procedure within 24 h

   (b) SMA thrombosis

   Perform embolectomy to SMA

   Assess flow

   If poor flow, saphenous vein graft (SVG) between infrarenal aorta and SMA

   (can use suprarenal aorta and pass graft behind pancreas to SMA)

   Administer postoperative heparin

   Resect nonviable segments and perform "second-look" procedure within 24 h

Common Curveballs

Patient had prior surgery

Patient has SMA embolus

Patient has SMA thrombosis

Patient has superior mesenteric vein (SMV) thrombosis

Patient needs preoperative resuscitation with or without SGC

Patient has necrotic bowel at second look

Patient has hypercoagulable syndrome

Patient had recent AAA repair with worry about graft contamination

Whole small bowel initially appears necrotic

How to identify SMA (elevate transverse colon, follow middle colic to SMA, will need to make incision in peritoneum of mesentery, artery is medial to SMV)

Patient returns 6 weeks after colonic ischemia was treated nonoperatively with stricture

Clean Kills

Performing anastomosis in setting of ischemia/contamination

Not performing second look if there is a question of viability

Not knowing how to deal with SMA embolus/thrombosis

Not resuscitating patient preoperatively but taking straight to OR

Discussing urokinase infusion for patient with embolic occlusion of mesenteric vessels or colonic ischemia

Delaying operation when patient is toxic

Not resecting necrotic bowel

Not understanding the difference between acute mesenteric ischemia and colonic ischemia

Colon Cancer

Concept

Colon cancer is the third most common cancer in the United States. Be prepared for unusual presentations of this malignancy (familial polyposis, invasion of surrounding structures, local recurrence, rising carcinoembryonic antigen (CEA) levels, metastases to the liver).

Way Question May Be Asked?

"A 54-year-old man presents to your office with a recent history of iron deficiency anemia. A recent colonoscopy performed by the referring gastroenterologist reveals a large adenomatous polyp in the cecum."

The vignette may also include symptoms such as a change in bowel habits, blood in stool, weight loss, abdominal pain, strong family history of colorectal cancer, a presentation similar to perforated diverticulitis, or even evidence of erosion into genitourinary system (fecaluria or pneumaturia).

How to Answer?

Take a complete history and perform a physical examination (may have been given all this already)

History
    Risk factors (family history, inflammatory bowel disease [IBD], previous polyps)
    Change in bowel habits
    Blood in stool
    Weight loss
    Pain
    Screening history

Physical examination
    Palpable abdominal masses
    Lymphadenopathy
    Palpable pathology on digital rectal examination/guaiac (+)

Diagnostic tests
    Usual laboratory tests (including CEA level, liver function tests [LFTs])
    Chest x-ray (CXR) or chest CT
    Colonoscopy (rule out synchronous lesions)
    ± Air-contrast barium enema
    ± CT of the abdomen/pelvis to rule out metastases (most would do this)

If patient was sent to you after a polypectomy, remember Haggit's classifications.

The patient needs resection in the following cases:
    Positive margin of resection
    Invading submucosa
    Poorly differentiated
    Venous/lymphatic invasion
    Cancer in any sessile polyp

Surgical Procedure

Do not forget mechanical/antibiotic bowel preparation (be prepared to discuss yours)

Consider preoperative ureteral stents for large/bulky/fixed tumor

"No touch" technique has never been proven to be of any clinical benefit

Resection includes the involved segment of colon along with its draining lymphatics and accompanying segmental blood supply both at their points of origin

Minimum 13 lymph nodes

Margins should be at least 5–10 cm

For tumors of the cecum and ascending colon, perform a right hemicolectomy (ligation of ileocolic, right colic, right branch of middle colic, removal of 5–8 cm of ileum to proximal transverse colon).

For tumors of the proximal transverse colon, perform an extended right hemicolectomy (ligation of ileocolic vessels to middle colic artery, removal of terminal ileum to splenic flexure, anastomosis between ileum and descending colon).

For tumors of the splenic flexure and descending colon, perform a left hemicolectomy (ligation of left colic with removal of descending colon and splenic flexure with anastomosis of transverse to upper sigmoid).

For tumors of the sigmoid and rectosigmoid, perform sigmoid colectomy (ligation of IMA distal to takeoff of left colic, anastomosis between descending colon and upper rectum).

For synchronous or metachronous cancers, perform a subtotal colectomy (removal of terminal ileum and ascending, transverse and descending colon with ileo sigmoid or ileorectal [if sigmoid resected] anastomosis); this is also indicated for patients with a proximal colon perforation due to an obstructing distal cancer.

For a tumor invading into adjacent organs, perform an en bloc resection, which does not preclude resection for cure or marking margins of resection with clips for postoperative radiotherapy (T4 but still stage IIB lesion if lymph nodes are negative). Check to make sure no other metastatic disease is present before proceeding (intraoperative examination and ultrasound of liver).

> If trigone of bladder is involved, perform cystectomy and ileal conduit.
>
> If invading head of pancreas, perform a Whipple procedure.
>
> If kidney is involved, check intravenous pyelogram to ensure the other kidney is okay before nephrectomy.

Malignant obstruction

1. Obstructing right-sided lesions: segmental resection with primary anastomosis
2. Obstructing left-sided lesions: diverting colostomy ± segmental resection
3. Perform primary resection with anastomosis and on-table lavage through the appendiceal stump and sterilized anesthesia tubing, with or without defunctioning stoma (not the conservative answer the board likes!)
4. Subtotal colectomy
5. Stenting is a treatment option for obstructing left-sided lesions prior to definitive operative management

For any obstructing lesion, clinical conversion of obstruction to near obstruction through NGT, intravenous fluid (IVF), and bowel rest should be attempted. If accomplished, prepare the bowel and perform the indicated segmental resection.

Perforated lesions

1. Perforated left colon cancer: segmental resection with end colostomy (Hartmann procedure)
2. Perforated right colon cancer: right hemicolectomy with primary anastomosis ± diverting stoma
3. Perforated cecum and obstructing left colon cancer:
   (a) If stable, then perform subtotal colectomy with primary ileorectal anastomosis
   (b) If unstable, then perform cecectomy, ileostomy, and mucous fistula; patient will need staged second operation to remove tumor

Liver lesions

Criteria for resection include the following:

1. Primary tumor can be completely resected
2. There are no other extrahepatic tumors aside from the primary
3. It is possible to resect all metastases in the liver while leaving enough hepatic remnant to maintain adequate liver function postoperatively, with 1-cm margins desirable

Adjuvant Treatment

Positive lymph nodes (stage III patients), invasion of other organs or distal metastases

5-FU and leucovorin is the treatment of choice for high-risk stage II and stage III disease

T4 lesion: radiotherapy to tumor bed to decrease local recurrence

Always consider adjuvant therapy in colon cancer patients with bowel obstruction, perforation, high-grade lymphatic/vascular involvement, and inadequate resection of regional lymph nodes.

Common Curveballs

Patient is sent to you after a polypectomy (what histology gets further surgery?)

Cancer presents as a large bowel obstruction

Cancer presents as perforated diverticulitis (be careful to check the frozen section intraoperatively and perform a wide resection if there is suspicion of cancer)

Cancer is eroding into surrounding structures (bladder, kidney, duodenum)

Cancer recurs locally

CEA rises in first year postoperatively

There is a peripheral lesion in the liver

If the patient has an 8-cm AAA this needs to be treated first then the near obstructing colon lesion; if the AAA is 5-cm then the near obstruction colon mass should be treated before the AAA repair.

Patient has IBD

There is a ureteral injury during dissection

There is bleeding from spleen after mobilizing the splenic flexure

There is a duodenal/vena cava injury when mobilizing right colon

There are synchronous lesions

Patient had prior colon surgery

Patient had a recent MI

Patient is unstable intraoperatively

Determining appropriate treatment with adjuvant chemotherapy

There is a postoperative anastomotic bleed, anastomotic leak, enterocutaneous fistula, or wound infection (could even be necrotizing—scenario switch)

Examiner asks you to describe the Duke's classification system

Examiner asks if you do your own colonoscopies (answer is yes!)

Pathologic specimen has less than 12 lymph nodes

Clean Kills

Forgetting colonoscopy to rule out synchronous lesions

Not performing preoperative staging workup

Not performing the correct surgical resection

Not performing en bloc resection when cancer has spread to adjacent organs

Talking about virtual colonoscopy

Forgetting bowel preparation

Radiofrequency liver ablation of resectable metastatic tumors

Performing liver resection (or major en bloc resection) while leaving extrahepatic (or other) disease behind

Summary

The definitive treatment for colon cancer is surgical resection. It is important to know the operative details of various segmentectomies because staging and adjuvant chemotherapeutic treatment options are dependent on adequate lymphovascular resection. The extent of segmental resection with or without anastomosis/stoma creation depends on the presentation of the tumor. Resection of liver metastases must be considered in patients without any identifiable extrahepatic tumors.

Enterocutaneous Fistula

Concept

Remember the FRIEND mnemonic: foreign body, radiation injury, ischemia/IBD, epithelialized tract, neoplasm, and distal obstruction are causes for fistula. Important concepts surrounding enterocutaneous fistulae are controlling infection and drainage, maximizing nutrition/electrolytes, and ruling out distal obstruction/associated abscess.

Way Question May Be Asked?

"A 43-year-old woman had an exploratory laparotomy with extensive enterolysis and adhesiolysis and repair of multiple enterotomies for persistent partial small bowel obstruction (PSBO). She develops a fever of 100.8°F. On examination, she has erythema and tenderness around the lower portion of her incision."

The question typically is open-ended, first with a discussion about how to manage a postoperative fever. It then hones in on small bowel contents coming out of the incision the next day (scenario switch).

How to Answer?

First, discuss the basic approach to postoperative fever, which must be systematic (remember the five *Ws* wind, wound, water, walking, wonder drugs).

History

    Atelectasis

    Urinary tract infection

    Intravenous (IV) sites

    Deep venous thrombosis/pulmonary embolism

    Wound infection

    Anastomotic leak

    Drug fever

    Rare entities (parotitis in patient who is nil per os [NPO] for a long period of time; acalculous cholecystitis, *Clostridium difficile*, transfusion reaction, thyroid storm, Addisonian crisis)

    Symptoms of cough, abdominal pain, shortness of breath, pain at IV sites

Physical examination

    Perform a close examination of wound for erythema, fluid, subcutaneous (SQ) air, and tenderness. Culture any drainage. Take out staples early.

Diagnostic Tests

    Laboratory tests

    CXR

    AXR

    Urinalysis (U/A), culture and sensitivity (C+S)

    Blood cultures (BCx)

    Ultrasound of abdomen/extremity

    CT scan

    Start antibiotics if there is evidence of sepsis.

    Once you have proven to the examiner that you understand how to workup postoperative fever, then the question will likely focus on management of the enterocutaneous fistula:

    Drain fistula with sump drain and protect surrounding skin

    Measure output of fistula (gives you information about likelihood of closure)

    Place central venous pressure (CVP) line and restore electrolytes and intravascular volume

    NPO, total parenteral nutrition (TPN)

    H_2 blockers

    Somatostatin (± any real benefit)

    Antibiotics if there is associated cellulitis/sepsis

    CT scan to rule out abscess and/or place percutaneous drain

    Fistulogram after 7–10 days to rule out distal obstruction

    Based on the fistulogram, there are one of two possibilities:

    1. No distal obstruction or intestinal discontinuation: Most enterocutaneous fistulae will close within 6 weeks

2. Distal obstruction, failure to close, or high-output fistula: Need operative repair involving taking down the fistula, bowel resection, and reanastomosis ± gastrostomy or jejunostomy feeding tube if prolonged postoperative ileus is suspected

Common Curveballs

Patient has SQ emphysema on examination of the wound, in which case the whole focus now shifts to managing a necrotizing soft-tissue infection

Patient has associated intra-abdominal abscess that cannot be percutaneously drained

There is a complication after placing CVP line (make sure you check CXR)

CT scan shows multiple fluid collections but no discrete abscess (always describe how you would order CT scan— "with IV/PO contrast")

Fistula fails to close and/or there is recurrence after bowel resection

Patient tries to push you into earlier operation

There is skin breakdown at the fistula site

Patient has a history of Crohn's disease

There is another fistula after you reoperate and take down the first enterocutaneous fistula

Having a discussion about TPN (1 g/kg/day protein, 25 kcal/kg/day carbohydrates)

(25 % glucose, 3–4 % amino acids, 10 % free fatty acids [FFA]; want 50 % of non-protein calories as glucose and 50 % as FFA)

Clean Kills

Failure to do standard fever workup

Operating too early for low-output fistula (give TPN chance to allow fistula to close)

Failure to consider all possible causes (such as distal obstruction) prior to reoperation

Starting a long discussion about the use of fibrin glue to close fistula tract

Failure to be methodical in the care of fistula: resuscitation, controlling fistula, expectant management, and supplemental nutrition/TPN

Hemorrhoids

Concept

Patients with hemorrhoids usually present with pain or bleeding. You need to recognize the difference between internal and external hemorrhoids. Know the various stages. Treatment is always initially conservative.

Way Question May Be Asked?

"A 25-year-old man presents to your office with the complaint of a thrombosed hemorrhoid. It occurred about 4 days ago and hurts whenever he sits down or has a bowel movement."

The patient may also present with rectal bleeding, acute thrombosis, or incontinence.

How to Answer?

Do not forget your basic history and physical examination or it will turn out to be something other than hemorrhoids.

History
  Constipation
  Pain
  Bleeding
  Topical therapy
  History of rectal complaints
  Family history of IBD
  Prolapse history
  Incontinence
Physical Examination
  Examine abdomen
  Rectal examination
  Anoscopy (with patient in left lateral decubitus position)
  Rigid sigmoidoscopy
  May need to do examination under anesthesia
  Look for malignancy, fistula, and other rectal pathology (careful for scenario switch!)
How to Answer
  Know the stages of internal hemorrhoids (above dentate line and therefore usually painless)
    I   Painless rectal bleeding
    II Prolapse with defecation, spontaneously reduce
    III Same as II, but reduction only manually
    IV Unable to reduce
  External hemorrhoids are below the dentate line and hurt when they become thrombosed.
  Nonoperative therapy
    4–6 weeks
    Bulk agents
    Increasing water intake (6–8 glasses/day)
    Topical agents (Tucks, Anusol HC, or Analpram)
    Sitz baths

Surgery

For acute thrombosis, bleeding thrombosis, and thrombosis with superficial necrosis, perform elliptical surgical excision under local anesthesia in your office.

For stage I and II internal hemorrhoids, perform rubber band ligation. Make sure there is not significant external disease or any other benign anorectal disease.

Banding of only one or two quadrants

No banding if patient has any prostheses (heart valve, breast implant, pacemaker, joint replacement)

Stage III and IV and recurrent symptomatic external hemorrhoids are treated with Ferguson closed hemorrhoidectomy (elliptical incision over each hemorrhoid down to sphincter and closure incorporating some of sphincter fibers to prevent prolapse)

Can also include lateral internal sphincterotomy

Make sure to inject perineum, submucosa, and pudendal nerves

Tape buttocks apart

Excise most symptomatic quadrant first

Excise minimal anoderm (risk of stenosis)

Common Curveballs

Patient has anal carcinoma

Patient has rectal prolapse rather than prolapsing hemorrhoid

Patient has anal fissure

Patient has postoperative incontinence or anal stenosis

Patient has a history of portal hypertension or is on blood thinners

Patient is older than 40 years (need to rule out proximal disease with barium enema (BE) or colonoscopy before instituting therapy)

Patient develops postbanding bleeding or infection

Patient has internal prostheses and desires hemorrhoidal banding

Patient has inflammatory bowel disease (no hemorrhoidectomy!)

Patient is pregnant (manage nonoperatively)

Patient has postoperative urinary retention, bleeding, or infection after closed hemorrhoidectomy

Clean Kills

Operating on thrombosed hemorrhoid after 48 h

Operating on stage I or II internal hemorrhoids

Not trying local measures first

Discussing the new Procedure for Prolapse and Hemorrhoids therapy

Not being able to deal with complications of the procedure you choose

Operating on patient with IBD

Not recognizing other anorectal pathology (cancer)

Incarcerated Hernia

Concept

Incarcerated hernia has multiple etiologies, but always remember the most common: hernias and adhesions. Do not forget the possibility of a malignancy, such as an obstructing proximal colon cancer and an incompetent ileocecal valve. It is important to decide in your own mind how long you will manage a small bowel obstruction (SBO) nonoperatively and what you will do intraoperatively with any compromised or nonviable small bowel.

Way Question May Be Asked?

"A 63-year-old woman was evaluated in the emergency department (ED) for a vomiting and abdominal distension. AXR reveals multiple air/fluid levels. What do you want to do?"

The question may be asked with a more subtle picture of SBO, or it may jump right into a discussion of management decisions. Do not spend too much time on history and physical examination if your examiner does not want you to.

How to Answer?

History

Pain

Distension

Previous abdominal surgery

Nausea/vomiting

Physical Examination

Vital signs (dehydration, fever)

Full examination, especially checking for hernias

Hyperactive bowel sounds

Peritoneal signs

Diagnostic Tests

Full laboratory tests (elevated white blood cells [WBC] of peritonitis)

AXR (three views, look at gas pattern)

CT scan (IV/PO contrast)

± Small bowel follow through (SBFT) in cases of PSBO that persist over 48 h

Surgical Treatment

1. NGT/NPO/IVF (always!)
2. Serial labs/examinations
3. Volume resuscitation (remember third space losses into gastrointestinal tract!)
4. Peritoneal signs or suggestion of hernia strangulation indicate surgery
   (a) Surgery for incarcerated hernia can be performed through an preperitoneal or traditional inguinal approach.
   (b) If you cannot reduce an incarcerated femoral hernia, divide the inguinal ligament; if strangulated, control strangulated contents and make lower midline incision.
   (c) Make sure to control sac and open under direct vision.
   (d) If the contents of the hernia drop into the abdominal cavity, explore either through preperitoneal incision by opening peritoneum or using laparoscope.
   (e) Do not use mesh in situations with possible ischemia.
   (f) If the hernia contents are ischemic, try the following:
       Warm packs over the area and come back after the hernia is repaired.
       If it is still ischemic, resect with primary anastomosis.

Common Curveballs

Hernia is incarcerated/strangulated
Hernia reduces with induction of general anesthesia
Need to divide inguinal ligament to free femoral hernia
Need to perform bowel resection
PSBO fails nonoperative management
Examiner asks you to describe inguinal anatomy
Not able to use mesh (know at least one non-mesh repair)
Patient has sliding hernia
SBFT/CT scan does not identify point of obstruction
Patient has malignancy

Clean Kills

Trying to perform laparoscopically (only do this if you have fellowship training in transabdominal preporitoneal hernia repair (TAPPs), but even then it is a risky answer!)
Not placing NGT or volume resuscitating patient
Not dividing inguinal ligament to free incarcerated femoral hernia
Not performing bowel resection for obviously ischemic bowel
Not knowing how to describe any non-mesh hernia repairs

Getting into discussion of using absorbable mesh (Surgissis or Alloderm) in a contaminated field with necrotic bowel
Not inspecting bowel that was incarcerated

Appendicitis

Concept

Appendicitis is one of the most common issues that general surgeons encounter. It affects almost 10 % of the population at some point during their lifetimes, with a peak occurrence between the ages of 10 and 30 years. In adults, the appendix has no function. Acute appendicitis is due to the obstruction of the lumen, which can be caused by either stool or lymphoid hyperplasia.

Way Question May Be Asked?

"A 16-year-old boy presents to the ED with a complaint of periumbilical pain that began yesterday, followed by nausea. He now states that the pain is worse in his right lower abdomen. What do you want to do?"

You will likely be asked if you want any other studies, such as a CT scan.

How to Answer?

History
    PQRST method for pain assessment (periumbilical pain that migrates to right lower quadrant [RLQ])
    Nausea/vomiting
    Appetite (common to have anorexia)
Physical Examination
    Fever
    Tenderness to palpation RLQ (McBurney's point) with possible voluntary guarding
    Rovsing sign—pain in RLQ with palpation of left lower quadrant (LLQ)
    Obturator sign—pain in RLQ on internal rotation of right hip
    Psoas sign—pain in RLQ with extension of the right hip

Data

Leukocytosis
CT scan—Appendicitis is a clinical diagnosis. However, because of how most hospital systems currently function, it is likely that a CT will be ordered prior to surgical evaluation. A CT scan is 95 % accurate at diagnosing

appendicitis. On CT, you will see an appendix >7 mm, wall thickening with enhancement, possible appendicolith, possible periappendiceal fat stranding, edema, fluid, phlegmon, or abscess.

Ultrasound—Sensitivity 90 %, specificity 80–90 %, appendix >7 mm, thick wall, non-compressible lumen, possible target sign or appendicolith

Surgical Treatment

NPO

IVF

IV antibiotics

Laparoscopic appendectomy: Use a 5-mm periumbilical port, 5-mm suprapubic port, and 12 mm LLQ port. Trace tinea of the right colon down to the base of the appendix. Make a window between the base of the appendix and mesoappendix. You can divide the mesoappendix with a stapler, Ligasure, or harmonic and the appendix with a stapler or endoloops. Remove appendix in an endobag through the 12-mm port, which should be closed at the facial layer.

Open appendectomy: Perform through a RLQ or midline incision. Trace tinea of right colon down to the base of the appendix. A window is made between the appendix and mesoappendix. Clamps and ties are used to divide the mesoappendix. A heavy absorbable tie is also used to tie the appendix at its base. It is clamped above and resected. The stump is then inverted with an absorbable Z-stitch and the wound is closed primarily.

If the base of the appendix is necrotic, a partial cecectomy is warranted.

If the patient has a perforated appendix with an abscess and is afebrile with a normal white count and no peritoneal signs, the patient is a candidate for CT-guided drainage of the abscess followed by interval appendectomy (especially for children).

If you find a normal appendix, look for a Meckle's or other cause of the pain. The appendix should be removed. Studies show that the morbidity from the procedure is so low, and it takes the appendix out of the equation if the patient ever has pain again.

If the patient is pregnant, appendicitis is the most common non-obstectrical surgical disease of the abdomen during pregnancy. It may be difficult to diagnose because of the similar symptoms of nausea, vomiting, and leukocytosis. In addition, after the fifth month, the fetus displaces the cecum and appendix upward. Ultrasound and magnetic resonance imaging (MRI) can be useful.

If the pathology comes back positive for a mucinous or carcinoid tumor, then consider the following:

1. Mucinous tumors are the most common tumor of the appendix. If the base of the appendix is involved, the patient will need a right hemicolectomy.
2. Carcinoid: If it is less than 1 cm and in tip, no further surgery is indicated.

   If it is greater than 2 cm or the base is involved, right hemicolectomy is indicated.

Common Curveballs

The patient is pregnant.

The appendix is normal but the ileum is inflamed, indicating that the patient probably has Crohn's disease. What do you do with the appendix? As long as the base is not involved, take it out.

There is a large phlegmon involving the right lower quadrant and you cannot identify the appendix. What do you do? Ileocectomy or full right hemicolectomy can be performed if needed.

The final pathology comes back with a mucinous or carcinoid tumor.

Clean Kills

Missing the diagnosis

Not taking the patient to the OR for anyone other than a patient with a perforated appendix who fits the criteria for an interval appendectomy

Not looking for another cause for the pain such as a Meckel's if the appendix is normal

Not knowing what to do if the patient has Crohn's disease

Not knowing what to do if the pathology comes back with a tumor

Summary

Patients with appendicitis typically present with periumbilical pain that migrates to the RLQ associated with nausea, anorexia, fever, and leukocytosis. Although appendicitis is a clinical diagnosis, most patients will already have a CT scan prior to surgical evaluation in the emergency room setting. Findings on the CT scan may include an appendicolith, appendix >7 mm, wall thickening and enhancement, periappendiceal fat stranding, fluid, phlegmon, or abscess. The appropriate treatment in the majority of cases is prompt laparoscopic or open appendectomy. The surgeon should also be aware of many complicating factors mentioned in the chapter because not all appendectomies are simple.

Intestinal Angina

Concept

Intestinal angina is caused by chronic occlusion of two of the three main visceral arteries (celiac, SMA, IMA). Post-prandial pain is related to insufficient blood flow 15–60 min after meals.

Way Question May Be Asked?

"A 69-year-old man with a history of peripheral vascular disease presents with weight loss and post-prandial abdominal pain."

Do not expect a clear description of "food fear" or weight loss. Many patients actually develop eating habits to avoid the post-prandial pain, including "small meal syndrome." The patient may even present with upper gastrointestinal dysmotility or ulcers.

How to Answer?

Complete history, including other types of vascular disease
Complete physical examination, including abdominal bruits
Be sure to ask about questions that relate to abdominal malignancy

Diagnostic Tests
  Cardiac workup (on all vascular patients)
  Visceral duplex showing stenosis (high-flow velocities) in celiac and SMA or reversal of flow in the hepatic artery
  Criterion standard: angiogram with anteroposterior and lateral views
  Endovascular techniques are an option for high-risk patients
  Be able to describe the operative technique:
Transabdominal approach through midline incision
Antegrade bypass from distal thoracic aorta
Bifurcated graft between the supraceliac aorta approached through the gastrohepaticomentum and both the celiac and the SMA
Bifurcated 12 × 7 mm graft
Left limb anastomosed to celiac trunk in end-to-side fashion, with heel on celiac trunk and toe as onlay path onto common hepatic artery
End-to-end bypass to SMA performed below the body of the pancreas
Aorta-SMA graft commonly placed behind the common hepatic artery

Must divide crus of right diaphragm to expose supraceliac aorta
Must divide ligament of Trietz to expose SMA infrapancreatically
Good communication with anesthesiologist before supraceliac clamping so as to permit adequate volume loading and unclamping for expected decrease in blood pressure
A retrograde bypass is another option from a healthy infrarenal aorta and the SMA distal to its occluded segment
You could also place a straight graft from infrarenal aorta to the SMA distal to its area of occlusion
IMA reconstruction increases postoperative morbidity
Follow patient with duplex ultrasound prior to hospital discharge and closely in the postoperative period (every 6 months)

Common Curveballs

You cannot get a mesenteric duplex at your hospital
Questions about surgical reconstruction of IMA
Patient has a bowel injury and cannot use an artificial graft
Patient has other pathology on initial exploratory laparotomy
Patient had prior abdominal surgery
Patient has postoperative graft thrombosis
Patient has acute MI
In workup for chronic mesenteric ischemia, patient develops acute mesenteric ischemia with bowel necrosis
Patient has postoperative hepatic or renal failure secondary to supraceliac aortic cross-clamp time (patient tolerance is typically less than 1 h)

Clean Kills

Not ruling out malignancy in patient with abdominal pain and weight loss
Not being able to describe operative technique
Not obtaining angiogram
Not performing appropriate preoperative workup/clearance in patient with obvious vascular disease

Large Bowel Obstruction

Concept

Large bowel obstruction has a broad DDx, with malignancy likely in the older population. History can be helpful here. You will probably be pushed into an operation on someone with obstruction secondary to malignancy or a diverticulitis-related stricture, or perhaps a patient that has even perforated secondary to their obstruction.

Way Question May Be Asked?

"A 61-year-old man is evaluated in the emergency room with recent constipation and change in bowel habits. He is complaining of sudden onset of diffuse abdominal pain/distension and has free air on AXR. What would you do?"

Be prepared to see an x-ray here.

How to Answer?

Have a DDx in your mind and work through it:
Obstructing cancer
Diverticular/ischemic stricture
Volvulus
Pseudo-obstruction (Ogilvie's)
Don't forget about history of prior operations

Physical Examination
   Examine abdomen
   Rectal examination, heme occult
   Rigid sigmoidoscopy (unless there are true peritoneal signs, it will have therapeutic value if volvulus)
Surgical Treatment
   If there are no signs of peritonitis:
      Gastrograffin enema
      CT scan of the abdomen
      NGT/Foley/IVF/NPO/serial exams
      Try to convert to near-obstructing lesion and perform semi-electively after bowel preparation
   If there are signs of peritonitis or complete obstruction:
      Surgery after initial evaluation and resuscitation (lines, IVF, antibiotics)
      In the OR:
      1. Perform a right hemicolectomy for obstructing lesions of right and proximal transverse colon (can do primary anastomosis here).
      2. Perform a left hemicolectomy/sigmoidectomy with colostomy and mucus fistula/Hartman's pouch for lesions obstructing distal transverse colon, left colon, or sigmoid.
      3. Perform a subtotal colectomy with primary anastomosis for obstructing lesion in left/sigmoid with perforation of cecum. This is useful in patients with metachronous lesions that are found after a previous resection for patients with synchronous cancers, but is not a good option in an unstable patient given the time involved.

4. Perform a right hemicolectomy/ileostomy/mucus fistula for an unstable patient with obstructing sigmoid/rectal lesion with perforation of cecum and gross contamination. The patient will then need work-up for malignancy and a second operation to remove disease if he survives. (Be careful how close you together you put stomas unless you want a situation where the appliance will never seal!).
5. Perform a defunctioning stoma (transverse loop colostomy) and then a later operation to remove obstructing tumor/mass in descending colon/sigmoid.

Common Curveballs

Patient has signs of peritonitis
There is perforation of right colon with mass on left
Rigid sigmoidoscopy does not find the cause of obstruction
Patient is unstable intraoperatively
Patient has AAA
Patient develops postoperative abscess or abdominal compartment syndrome
Patient develops ischemia at colostomy site
Patient becomes coagulopathic during the operation
TherInability to pass rectal tube for volvulus or keep in place to give patient bowel prep
Cecum is overdistended in follow-up of pseudo-obstruction or perforates
Distal cancer is fixed to pelvic structures
Ureter/duodenal/liver injury occurs while mobilizing right colon
Splenic injury occurs while mobilizing splenic flexure
Hard peripheral liver lesion is identified at time of emergency operation for peritonitis
Patient had prior abdominal/colonic surgery

Clean Kills

Doing anastomosis in face of frank contamination
Not knowing how to contruct ileostomy/mucus fistula/Hartman pouch
Talking about on-table bowel lavage
Performing long operation in elderly/unstable patient
Using *barium* enema rather than *water-soluble* contrast when concerned about cause of obstruction and possible perforation
Discussing colonoscopically placed stents for malignant obstruction (an option, but the risk of perforation is high)
Getting a CT scan on a patient with peritonitis
Discussing cecostomy tubes or IV neostigmine

Lower GI Bleeding

Concept

Lower GI bleeding (LGIB) has a broad DDx, but three common pathologies need to be ruled out: diverticulosis, angiodysplasia, and cancer. LGIB is likely to be self-limited in more than 80 % of patients. Rebleeding is more common with arteriovenous malformation (AVM) than diverticular disease unless the patient is young. Approximately 10 % of patients will require surgical intervention.

Way Question May Be Asked?

"A 69-year-old woman is seen in the ED for dizziness after abruptly moving her bowels and producing a large amount of maroon-colored stools. She is tachycardic to the 110s, but her blood pressure is stable. What do you want to do?"

It is important to determine early in your mind if the patient is stable or unstable and have a plan for transfusion. The scenario is likely to be pretty basic because the examiner wants to get to your management algorithm and your indications for surgery. Focus your algorithm around three points: hemodynamic stabilization, localization, and site-specific intervention.

How to Answer?

Have a DDx in your mind and work through it:
Diverticulosis (painless bleeding)—by far the most common etiology
Angiodysplasia (painless bleeding)
Cancer
Ischemia
IBD
Infectious
Anorectal pathology
Small bowel pathology (tumor, Meckel's diverticulum)
    Do not forget about brisk bleeding from an upper GI source causing rapid transit (proximal to the ligament of Treitz)
History (obtained during initial resuscitation)
    Age (<30 years: consider IBD or Meckel's, >30 years: diverticular diagnosis, with AVM most common)
    Previous surgery (e.g. prior AAA repair or resection for diverticular disease/cancer)
    Medications/known coagulopathy (nonsteroidal anti-inflammatory drugs [NSAIDS], aspirin (ASA), Coumadin, Plavix, Lovenox, Pradaxa)

Prior bleeding episodes
Trauma
Radiation (ischemia)
Pain with bleeding episode or tenesmus
Amount of bleeding, color
Bruisablility
Dizziness or other evidence of shock
Physical Examination
    Vital signs (Orthostatic, tachycardic, tachypneic)
    Signs of liver disease (telangiectasias, thrombocytopenia, coagulopathy)
    Examine abdomen (prior scars)
    Rectal examination
    Necessary parts of physical examination:
        Placing NGT—gastric lavage
        Bloody=esophagogastroduodenoscopy (EGD), clear=EGD/colonoscopy, bilious=colonoscopy
        Anoscopy
        Rigid sigmoidoscopy (to rule out rectal source)
Diagnostic Tests
    Full laboratory panel, including complete blood count, prothrombin time/partial thromboplastin time, followed with serial hemoglobin levels
    Tagged red blood cell (RBC) scan (detects bleeding of 0.1–0.4 ml/min)—Sensitive
    Angiography (detects bleeding of 1–1.5 ml/min and can be therapeutic via vasopressin infusion/embolization)—Specific
    Colonoscopy (useful after preparation in those patients who do not require urgent operation)

Surgical Treatment

1. Know when to go perform surgery:
   Transfusion of >4 U packed RBC in 24 h
   LGIB that causes hypotension
   LGIB that is refractory to maximal medical therapy
   Continuous bleeding without identifiable source after 72 h
   Rebleeding within 1 week of initial episode
2. After tagged RBC scan:
   (a) If positive and patient is unstable, proceed to surgery. If patient is stable, proceed with immediate angiogram.
   (b) If negative, you can still repeat within 24 h and prepare for colonoscopy.
3. After angiogram:
   (a) If positive, administer vasopressin 0.2 U/min to control bleeding (no embolization of colonic pathology!)
   (b) If negative, prepare for colonoscopy unless unstable (then surgery)

Provocative angiography (preoperative)—short-acting anticoagulants allow for methylene blue injection with subsequent immediate operative intervention

The order of vessel evaluation is as follows: SMA injected first, then IMA, followed by celiac trunk if the first two are negative.

4. If you can identify the source, then perform segmental resection.
5. If you cannot identify source:
   (a) Provocative angiography
   (b) Subtotal colectomy with primary ileorectal anastomosis or ileostomy depending on the patient's stability
   (c) If you see blood in mid-ileum or above, consider a small bowel source prior to subtotal colectomy

Common Curveballs

Entire colon is filled with blood on colonoscopy

On colonoscopy, there is blood in the terminal ileum

There is colonic infarction after an attempt at angiographic embolization of diverticular bleed

You have to operate on the patient before RBC scan or angiogram

Being asked when it is appropriate to perform

tagged RBC scan, angiography, and colonoscopy, as well as the advantages/disadvantages of each

Management of the unstable patient preoperatively or intraoperatively

Patient requires continued transfusion (what is your threshold for taking patient to the OR?)

No source is identified preoperatively or intraoperatively

A ureter, duodenal, or liver injury occurs while mobilizing right colon

Splenic injury occurs when mobilizing splenic flexure

Hard peripheral liver lesion is identified at the time of emergency operation

Patient had prior abdominal/colonic surgery

Patient had recent MI or has severe cardiac disease

Patient has an upper GI source (scenario switch)

Patient is taking NSAIDS, aspirin, Plavix, Coumadin, Pradaxa, or Lovenox

Patient has bleeding from stoma after subtotal colectomy

Patient is a Jehovah's Witness and will not accept blood transfusions

Patient has acquired immunodeficiency syndrome

Clean Kills

Embolizing colonic lesion identified by arteriogram

Not placing NGT (failing to consider upper GI source)

Not performing rigid sigmoidoscopy

Not ruling out/correcting coagulopathy (Coumadin, ASA, liver disease, Plavix, Lovenox)

Performing a long operation in an elderly/unstable patient

Not performing subtotal colectomy when you cannot identify the source

Sending an unstable patient for a bleeding scan

Not considering an angiogram or bleeding scan but proceeding straight to surgery

Not examining the terminal ileum or performing EGD if the source is not found on colonoscopy

Any delay in resuscitative measures

Summary

To correctly diagnose and treat LGIB, a multidisciplinary approach must be taken. A well-developed algorithm focused on hemodynamic stabilization, localization, and site-specific intervention is key to successful treatment. Surgical intervention is the therapy of choice in unstable patients refractory to resuscitation or when all other treatment modalities have failed. Diverticular disease is the most common culprit.

Perirectal Abscess

Concept

Perirectal abscess is characterized by constant pain in the rectal area. It arises from an infected anal gland. After drainage, about half of patients will develop an anal fistula.

Way Question May Be Asked?

"A 50-year-old man presents the ED with the complaint of hemorrhoids. It started about 3 days ago, and the patient complains of constant severe pain and low-grade fever and chills."

How to Answer?

Take a full history and physical examination.

History
  Constipation
  Pain just with defecation (fissure) or constant (abscess)
  Bleeding
  Topical therapy
  History rectal complaints (incontinence, etc.)
  Family history of IBD

Fever/chills

Prior rectal surgery

Human immunodeficiency virus (HIV) status

Physical examination

Examine abdomen

Rectal examination (patient in left lateral decubitus position!)

Anoscopy/sigmoidoscopy is not necessary

May need to do examination under anesthesia

Look for malignancy, fistula, and other rectal pathology (be careful for scenario switch!)

Diagnostic Tests

Laboratory work (elevated WBC)

CT scan of pelvis (may predict level of the abscess)

Types of Abscesses

I   Perianal—abscess in SQ tissue adjacent to the anal verge

II   Ischiorectal—the infection travels through the sphincters into the ischiorectal space; may have minimal external signs, usually fluctuance a few centimeters from anal verge

III Intersphincteric—fluctuance/tenderness on rectal exam, abscess between internal and external sphincters

IV   Horseshoe—bilateral ischiorectal spaces involved and deep posterior anal space

V   Supralevator—from upward extension of intersphincteric or ischiorectal abscess, or from downward extension of pelvic process (diverticulitis, appendicitis, Crohn's disease)

Surgery

Immediate incision and drainage

For types I and II treatment is incision and drainage under regional or general anesthesia.

For type III, treatment is drainage into the anal canal.

For type IV, drain deep postanal space by dividing overlying internal sphincter and lower portion of external sphincter and making two counter incisions to drain ischiorectal extensions.

For type V, determine the source first. If pelvic pathology, then perform external drainage of abscess; if rectal source, then perform drainage with a mushroom catheter.

Avoid fistulotomy at time of abscess drainage

Low threshold to return to surgery if no improvement is seen (especially in supralevator abscesses)

May need diverting colostomy for severe/recurrent supralevator abscess

If scenario continues to management of fistula, surgery is always the answer:

Make sure to rule out associated GI diseases (IBD, HIV)

Know patient's baseline continence level prior to going to the OR

Evaluate entire colon with barium enema (BE) or colonoscopy

May need to inject H_2O_2 or methylene blue to identify openings

Fistulotomy unless fistula involves > 30 % sphincter fibers or is an anterior fistula in a female

Must assess the level at which the fistula traverses the sphincters

Treat intestinal disease in IBD, which will often accompany resolution of perianal disease or use Seton as a drain

Liberal use of the Seton (a nonabsorbable suture or rubber band placed through the tract that stimulates scar formation, gradually cuts through the sphincter mechanism as it is tightened over next several weeks, and minimizes incontinence)

Goodsall's Rule:

When the external line lies anterior to the transverse anal line, the track runs in a direct radial line to the internal opening in the anal canal.

When the external opening is posterior to the transverse anal line, the track curves backward to the posterior midline.

Common Curveballs

Patient has anal/rectal cancer

Patient develops postoperative anal fistula

Patient has HIV

Patient has postoperative incontinence

Patient has history of portal hypertension or is on blood thinners

Patient has inflammatory bowel disease

Patient is pregnant

Unable to perform rectal examination in office/ED (examination under anesthesia)

Patient has a severe abscess that does not improve despite drainage (may need colostomy)

Clean Kills

Not recognizing the scenario and mistaking it for thrombosed hemorrhoid

Performing a fistulotomy during the first treatment of anal abscess

Admitting patient, placing on IV antibiotics, and "waiting" for abscess to mature/reach the surface

Not recognizing associated GI diseases

Not ruling out pelvic pathology with supralevator abscess
Not making counter incisions with horseshoe abscess
Not knowing Goodsall's rule
Not knowing how/when to use a Seton

Rectal Cancer

Concept

The prognosis for rectal cancer is worse than for colon cancer stage for stage. Preoperative therapy is offered to most patients except those with disease limited to the mucosa. Examiners will likely push you to understand when you will perform low anterior resection (LAR), abdominoperineal resection (APR), or transanal excision.

Way Question May Be Asked?

"A 62-year-old woman with a history of painless rectal bleeding presents to your office for evaluation. On digital rectal examination, she has a fixed, ulcerated mass beginning at 5 cm. What do you want to do?"

You may also be presented with a patient that has an obstruction, pain, or bright red blood per rectum.

How to Answer?

History
  Risk factors (family history, previous pelvic irradiation, smoking status, use of alcohol/drugs)
  Pain
  Change in bowel habits
  Previous colorectal polyps or cancer
  Previous colorectal or genitourinary surgery
  Smoking status, use of alcohol/drugs
  Continence status (you do not want to do a restorative resection in a patient with high likelihood of postoperative incontinence)
Physical Examination
  Digital rectal examination (is the lesion fixed, relation of the lesion to the anal verge, size/circumference involved)
  Lymphadenopathy (perform fine needle aspiration on any groin nodes if enlarged)
  Rigid sigmoidoscopy (mobility of tumor and distance from anal verge)
Diagnostic Tests
  Biopsy!
  Full laboratory work (especially LFTs, CEA)

Fecal occult blood test
  CXR or chest CT (to rule out metastasis)
  Flexible sigmoidoscopy and colonoscopy (to evaluate the rest of colon)
  Endorectal ultrasound (depth of invasion and lymph node status)
  ± CT scan (utility is in determination of extrarectal extent of disease)
  ± Double-contrast barium enema
  ± MRI (may be endorectal)
  Newer modalities include virtual colonoscopy and stool DNA assays
  Positron emission tomography (PET) scanning has low yield in determining pelvic lymphatic metastases

Surgical Treatment

Who gets radical resection? (low anterior resection (LAR), abdominoperineal resection (APR))
  Remember, try to get 2–5 cm distal margins (<1 cm with adjuvant chemotherapy allows sphincter preservation). You must also have radial margins > 2 mm.
  Always perform total mesorectal excision.
  LAR is easiest for lesions in the upper third of the rectum.
  If trying for lesions >5 cm from anal verge, use colonic J-pouch with coloanal anastomosis.
  Creation of a diverting loop ileosotomy/colostomy for any anastomosis constructed within 5 cm of the anal verge is a technique to reduce the incidence of leak (reversed 8–12 weeks postoperatively after gastrograffin enema demonstrates no leak).
  Involved organs (e.g., uterus, adnexa, posterior vaginal wall, bladder) should be removed en bloc.
  APR should be strongly considered for all invasive rectal cancer < 5 cm from anal verge. Closure of pelvic peritoneum is not necessary. Consider posterior vaginectomy in women with anterior tumors. Have the patient marked by a stomal therapist preoperatively.
  High-risk patients can be treated with radiation and re-evaluation ± fulgeration.
Who gets local excision? (transanal, transanal endoscopic microsurgery [TEM], transrectal)
  Think mobile, nonulcerated lesion
No more than 4 cm in diameter, no more than one-third the circumference and < 8 cm from anal verge
  T1–2 N0 lesions
  Well to moderately differentiated tumors without ulceration
  No lymphatic invasion on endoscopic ultrasound
  Perform in prone-jackknife position and excise tumor with full thickness of rectal wall into perirectal fat with 1 cm circumferential margin

Make sure to check path: rule out invasion of muscularis, lymphovascular invasion, or poorly differentiated tumor

Orient carefully for pathologist

Follow up with digital rectal examination, CEA levels, proctoscopy, and transanal ultrasonography

May be offered as a palliative treatment (fulguration, endocavitary irradiation)

Who gets chemotherapy/radiotherapy (5-FU and levamisole)?

TNM staging is best determined by endorectal ultrasound and MRI with endorectal coil.

There is controversy regarding preoperative vs. postoperative radiation treatment: Preoperative treatment may reduce tumor burden (tattoo the area preoperatively because the tumor may "melt" away). Postoperative treatment allows for more accurate treatment of staged cancer.

If tumor is resectable, give adjuvant chemoradiation when tumor is T2 with clean margins after transanal excision (TAE) or whenever tumor is T3–4 or N1–2 or has positive margins after LAR/APR.

If tumor is unresectable, give adjuvant chemoradiation.

Give chemotherapy for resectable metastatic disease.

Newer agents are irinotecan and oxaliplatin.

Common Curveballs

Indications for local resection

Proper use of preoperative adjuvant therapy

Management of postoperative anastomotic leak, pelvic abscess

The technical details of an APR

Pathology after local excision illustrates stage II depth of invasion

Patient had prior colon surgery

Patient has IBD

Patient has local recurrence or positive margins after local transanal excision

Injury to the ureter occurs during LAR

Patient has postoperative sexual dysfunction

Management of presacral hemorrhage

Patient has stomal complications with APR (stenosis, retraction, hernia, prolapse)

There is invasion of the bladder/prostate/vagina

Utility of PET scanning

Clean Kills

Performing a local resection when not indicated

Treating anal cancer like rectal cancer

Not doing the staging workup preoperatively

Not evaluating rest of the colon preoperatively

Attempting the procedure laparoscopically (no randomized studies yet support this)

Summary

Before proceeding with the treatment of rectal cancer, it is important to correctly stage the tumor. Through a combination of various imaging modalities, the anatomy and location of the lesion and the type of pathology yielded from biopsy, the stage of the tumor can be determined and a treatment plan formulated. The indication for neoadjuvant chemoradiation treatment as well as the approach/type of surgery will be dictated by the stage of the tumor. Always take into account the patient's continence status before deciding on the type of operative procedure.

Right Lower Quadrant Pain

Concept

A wide variety of pathologies can contribute to RLQ pain. Much information can be gathered by the history and physical examination. Plan out a DDx in your head and ask appropriate questions. In the OR, be prepared for what to do if the appendix is negative.

Way Question May Be Asked?

"A 21-year-old woman is evaluated in the ED for RLQ pain. Her temperature is elevated and she has peritoneal signs. You explore the patient through a RLQ transverse incision and find a normal appendix. What do you want to do?"

You will likely be placed in the position of taking the patient to the OR and finding a normal appendix, then asked what to do next.

How to Answer?

History
  Character of pain
  GI/genitourinary symptoms
  Previous surgery
  Appetite
  Menstrual history (if female)
  Family history of IBD
Physical Examination
  Abdominal examination: tenderness, guarding, rebound, mass (pulsatile?)
  Rectal examination

Pelvic examination (if female)—do not trust someone else's examination!

Look for hernia

Diagnostic Tests

Full laboratory panel (including amylase and pregnancy test)

Urinalysis

Abdominal series

EKG/CXR (depending on patient age)

CT scan (in equivocal cases)

Ultrasound—transvaginal is helpful in females to rule out gynecologic processes

If unsure, it would be acceptable to admit patient overnight for observation (no antipyretics or antibiotics!)

Surgical Treatment

1. Appendicitis

   Describe typical resection

   If the base is necrotic, perform a partial cecectomy

   If there is an abscess, perform a CT-guided drain followed by interval appendectomy

   If it comes back carcinoid, perform a right hemicolectomy for the following:

   Carcinoid >1.5 cm

   Located at base of appendix

   Serosal involvement

   Positive lymph nodes

2. Ectopic pregnancy

   If unruptured, perform a salpingotomy, evacuate contents, and repair

   If ruptured, perform a salpingectomy (preserve ovary)

3. Tubovarian abscess (TOA)

   Appendectomy (so there is no future confusion)

   Lavage, drain

   Salpingo-oopherectomy if necrotic

   Can treat with antibiotics (ceftriaxone and doxycycline) if only pelvic inflammatory disease

4. Meckel's diverticulum

   If appendectomy is negative, make sure to examine the last 2 ft of terminal ileum

   For a wedge resection of diverticulum, you may need segmental resection with primary anastomosis depending on inflammation

   Always do an appendectomy before closing!

   If there is an incidental finding, remove if the patient is <18 years of age or there is a narrow neck to diverticulum

5. Terminal ileitis

   Perform an appendectomy if the base of appendix is free of disease

   Treat medically with azulfidine, prednisone, metronidazole

Surgery should be performed only for obstruction, bleeding, perforation, non-healing fistulas, and failure of medical management

6. Solid ovarian mass

   (a) Post-menopausal patient—resect with full staging for ovarian cancer (washings, biopsies, omentectomy, para-aortic lymph node sampling, total abdominal hysterectomy bilateral salphingo-oophorectomy (TAH/BSO))

   (b) Pre-menopausal patient—obtain washings, biopsies, frozen section after incisional biopsy; if malignant, perform a unilateral salpingo-oophorectomy

7. Cystic ovarian mass

   (a) Post-menopausal patient—follow ovarian cancer staging procedure

   (b) Pre-menopausal patient—treat as solid ovarian mass in pre-menopausal patient as described above if ≥5 cm; otherwise, follow with ultrasound and refer to gynecologist for follow-up

Common Curveballs

Any one of a variety of diagnoses, none of which are appendicitis

Be prepared for the scenario to switch right after you describe how to deal with one problem (e.g., after answering for Meckel's diverticulum, you may be asked, "Okay, what if the terminal ileum is inflamed?")

Changing scenarios will be the norm here

Other causes not listed above include the following:

Giardiasis

Renal stone

Diverticulitis (right or left sided ± abscess)

Leaking AAA (take to OR immediately)

Acute mesenteric ischemia

Incarcerated hernia

Testicular torsion/ovarian torsion

Ruptured ovarian cyst

Patient is pregnant (appendix may not be in pelvis depending on trimester)

Patient has HIV (cytomegalovirus enteritis, tuberculosis, lymphoma)

Mesenteric lymphadenitis

There is no problem in RLQ except bile staining and a mass in the right upper quadrant (perforated duodenal ulcer—scenario switch)

Clean Kills

Describing complicated laparoscopic procedures

Not looking for Meckel's diverticulum or into pelvis when appendix is normal

Not knowing what to do for carcinoid or Crohn's disease
Fumbling with the change in scenarios (can happen anytime)
Forgetting a pregnancy test in women of child-bearing age
Forgetting a pelvic examination in women
Not performing a rectal examination
Getting a CT scan showing appendicitis and discussing incidental appendectomy
Not having a broad DDx

Crohn's Disease

Concept

Crohn's disease is chronic transmural inflammation of the GI tract of an unknown etiology. It has a bimodal distribution, with the first peak occurring in the 20s to 30s and a second smaller peak in the 60s. It has a strong familial association and usually involves the small bowel and colon but can affect any part of the GI tract. Pathology includes the following: skip lesions, fat wrapping, apthous ulcers, cobblestoning, transmural inflammation, and non-caseating granulomas. Long-standing disease can lead to an increased risk of small bowel and colon cancer.

Way Question May Be Asked?

"A 25-year-old man presents a complaint of colicky intermittent abdominal pain that has been getting progressively worse and is associated with diarrhea. He is thin in appearance and states that he has been having trouble keeping his weight on. What do you want to do?"

How to Answer?

History
  Family history
  Previous episodes of abdominal pain and diarrhea
  Extraintestinal manifestations (present in 30 %): erythema multiform, erythema nodosum, pyodermagangrenosum, iritis, uveitis, conjunctivitis, arthritis, ankylosing spondylitis, sclerosing cholangitis
Physical Examination
  Vital signs (fever if any complications are present)
  Abdominal examination (tenderness vs. peritoneal signs)
  Rectal examination (usually spares rectum, but the patient may have perianal disease; check for fistulas)
Diagnostic Tests
  Full laboratory panels
  Barium study—can show cobblestoning, narrowing in the diseased area and fistulas

CT scan—will show thickening of the involved bowel, more useful when you suspect a potential complication of Crohn's such as obstruction or perforation
Endoscopy—can show the inflammation, ulcers, cobblestoning, biopsy can be obtained
Stool studies

Treatment

Medical treatment
  1. Sulfasalazine (most common treatment)
  2. Corticosteriods
  3. Antibiotics (especially metronidazole)
  4. Infliximab
Surgical treatment
  Surgical intervention should be directed specifically to the complications (obstruction and perforation) and only the involved bowel should be removed.
  Perform resection with primary anastomosis if the infection is controlled and the patient has good nutritional status. If there are signs of sepsis and the patient is malnourished, you can divert.
  Strictures—can be treated with strictureplasty instead of resection
  Fistulas demonstrated on x-ray but not of clinical consequence should not be treated

Common Curveballs

The patient presents with one of the complications of Crohn's disease
Examiner asks about the differences between Crohn's disease and ulcerative colitis (UC)
Examiner asks about the extraintestinal manifestations
Examiner asks about the medical treatment

Clean Kills

Not distinguishing between Crohn's disease and UC
Not ruling out infectious colitis or *C. difficile*
Not attempting medical therapy; surgery is reserved for complications of Crohn's disease only
Starting to talk about Remicade or steroids without really understanding their implications/side effects

Summary

Crohn's disease is a transmural inflammation of unknown etiology that can occur in any portion of the GI tract. Patients with Crohn's disease usually present with a

combination of abdominal pain, diarrhea, and weight loss. The typical pathological findings of Crohn's disease include transmural inflammation, fat wrapping, apthous ulcers, cobblestoning, and skip lesions. In addition, patients with Crohn's disease can also have a variety of extraintestinal manifestations that can be associated with the disease. The primary treatment for Crohn's disease is supportive and medical and surgical intervention is reserved for the complications.

Ulcerative Colitis

Concept

UC is an inflammatory bowel disease of unknown etiology. It affects the mucosa and submucosa but spares the muscularis of the rectum and colon. Rectal involvement is the hallmark of the disease. It does not have skip areas or full thickness involvement like Crohn's disease. Surgery is performed for intractable disease, toxic megacolon, massive bleeding, and dysplasia/carcinoma.

Way Question May Be Asked?

"A 25-year-old man presents to the ED with abdominal pain and bloody diarrhea. Physical examination reveals a temperature of 101°F, moderate abdominal tenderness, and moderate distension. What do you want to do?"

The presentation will usually include some form of diarrhea, abdominal pain, and fever. Rarely are arthritis, uveitis, and pyoderma mentioned. Make sure to differentiate the patient with ulcerative colitis flare from the patient with toxic megacolon!

How to Answer?

History
    Family history
    Extraintestinal manifestations (arthritis, ankylosing spondylitis, erythema nodosum, pyodermagangrenosum, primary sclerosing cholangitis (PSC)—everything except PSC will improve with colectomy)
    Medications (steroids?)
    Previous flares
Physical Examination
    Vital signs (fever, tachycardia, sepsis)
    Abdominal examination (peritonitis?)
    Rectal examination (will always be involved in UC)
Diagnostic Tests
    Full labs (leukocytosis)
    Sigmoidoscopy/colonoscopy (with biopsy if it is not an acute flare)

Abdominal series (colon dilatation, free air)
± CT scan
Stool for *C. difficile*, ova and parasites (O+P), enteric pathogens

Surgical Treatment

Surgical treatment is indicated for toxic megacolon, massive bleeding, intractable disease, and dysplasia/cancer.

1. If you suspect toxic megacolon
    (a) Intensive care unit with IVF and transfusion if necessary
    (b) Antibiotics
    (c) NGT/NPO/bowel rest
    (d) TPN
    (e) Steroids
    (f) Serial labs/x-rays/examinations
    (g) If there is failure to improve within 48 h or worsening examination, proceed to the OR for subtotal colectomy and Brooke ileostomy (can bring up mucous fistula to lower portion of wound and not open; it will open in approximately one-third of patients but it is less risky than rectal staple line leak)
    (h) In an unstable patient, you can perform the Turnbull procedure, diverting ileostomy and blowhole loop colostomy
2. If patient responds to medical treatment or has a less acute presentation:
    (a) Barium enema to evaluate extent of disease
    (b) Colonoscopy and multiple biopsies to evaluate for dysplasia
    (c) Upper GI series with SBFT (to rule out Crohn's disease) if any doubt
    (d) Medical treatment with:
        Aminosalicylates/mesalamine (most common medical treatment)
        Prednisone
        Steroid enemas
        6-Mercaptopurine
        Diphenoxylate/atropine
        Low-residue diet
    (e) Surgery is indicated for:
        UC that is unresponsive to medical therapy (uncontrolled diarrhea, failure to thrive in children)
        Dysplasia or cancer on colonoscopic biopsy
        Severe extracolonic disease
    (f) Surgical options include the following (choice depends on severity of rectal involvement):
        Total proctocolectomy with Brooke ileostomy (if severe)
Total colectomy, anorectal mucosectomy, and ileorectal pull-through anastomosis (use diverting ileostomy here)
Total proctocolectomy with continent ileostomy (Kock pouch)

Common Curveballs

UC presents as massive bleeding

Patient does not respond to medical treatment

Patient is unstable

There is free perforation

Patient has postoperative intraabdominal abscess

Patient has leak after ileoanal anastomosis

You are asked for your medical regimen for the chronic form of the disease

Scenario changes from toxic megacolon to a chronic form of UC

Examiner asks about the differences between UC and Crohn's disease

Examiner asks you to describe extracolonic manifestations

Staple line on Hartmann's pouch leaks

Patient with perirectal abscess/fistula has Crohn's disease (how will you manage?)

Clean Kills

Not making the diagnosis of UC

Not ruling out infectious diarrhea or *C. difficile* and taking out the entire colon

Not performing sigmoidoscopy

Not treating toxic megacolon with steroids, antibiotics, and serial examinations

Not differentiating from Crohn's disease

Not knowing the difference between UC and Crohn's disease

Summary

Ulcerative colitis is a form of inflammatory bowel disease of unknown etiology that usually occurs in the second to third decade of life and presents with abdominal pain and bloody diarrhea. UC differs from Crohn's disease in that it is not transmural but continuous, usually starting at the rectum. Similar to Crohn's disease, UC can present with extraintestinal manifestations. The primary treatment for UC is medical. However, over time, patients with UC have a high risk of developing cancer and should be closely monitored with colonoscopy and biopsies. The surgical indications for UC include toxic megacolon, massive bleeding, intractable disease, and dysphagia/carcinoma. The specific surgical procedure depends on the reason for the surgery and the stability of the patient but most frequently involves a total proctocolectomy.

Anna Goldenberg Sandau and Roy L. Sandau

Carcinoid

Concept

This malignant neuroendocrine tumor arises from enterochromatic-type Kulchitsky cells. The most common presentation is small bowel obstruction (SBO). It is otherwise asymptomatic unless it occurs outside of the gastrointestinal (GI) tract: bronchus, rectum, metastasis to liver so that hormones elaborated can bypass the portal system. The symptoms of flushing and diarrhea occur from excess blood serotonin levels. Approximately 80 % of carcinoid tumors are found within 2 ft of the ileocecal valve.

Way Question May Be Asked?

"A 31-year-old man undergoes a laparoscopic appendectomy for acute appendicitis and the pathology comes back with a 2.1 cm carcinoid at the base of the appendix. What do you do?"

"A patient with no previous surgery presents with a history of intermittent diarrhea, now with small bowel obstruction. Computed tomography (CT) scan shows liver metastasis."

How to Answer?

Treatment depends on three factors:
1. Size (<1 cm, 1–2 cm, >2 cm)
2. Site (appendix, rectum, duodenum)
3. Pathology (depth of invasion or lymph node involvement)

A.G. Sandau, D.O. (✉)
General Surgery, University of Medicine and Dentistry of New Jersey, School of Osteopathic Medicine, Stratford, NJ, USA
e-mail: agolde5044@yahoo.com

R.L. Sandau, D.O.
General Surgery, Kennedy University Hospital, 2201 Chapel Ave West, Suite 100, Cherry Hill, NJ 08002, USA

Appendix
1. <1 cm: Appendectomy
2. 1–2 cm: Ileocecectomy
3. >2 cm or positive lymph node (LN): Right hemicolectomy

Rectum
1. <1 cm: Endoscopic resection
2. 1–2 cm: Transrectal resection enucleation
3. >2 cm or positive LN: Abdominal peritoneal resection
   Jejunum or ileum: wide local excision with mesenteric lymph nodes

Duodenum
1. <1 cm: Endoscopic resection
2. 1–2 cm: Transduodenal enucleation or segmental resection
3. >2 cm or positive LN: Pancreaticoduodenectomy

Liver Metastases
1. Enucleation, multiple resections, or lobectomy
2. Selective embolization
3. Radiofrequency ablation

Medical Therapy
1. Symptomatic carcinoid tumors: Somatostatin and interferon-α for palliating symptoms
2. Advanced cases: Chemotherapy with streptozotocin, doxorubicin, and 5-FU

Preoperative workup:
1. Confirmatory diagnostic testing: 24-h urine for 5-hydroxyindoleacetic acid levels and chromogranin A levels
2. Somatostatin receptor scintography (octreotide scan) for localization
3. Computed tomography (CT) angiogram for liver and lymph node involvement
   Postoperative surveillance: Chromogranin A levels

M.A. Neff (ed.), *Passing the General Surgery Oral Board Exam*,
DOI 10.1007/978-1-4614-7663-4_4, © Springer Science+Business Media New York 2014

Carcinoid crisis may occur shortly after inducing anesthesia with the following:

Cardiac arrhythmias

Labile blood pressure

Generalized flushing

Treatment with octreotide

In carcinoid syndrome:

Only 10 % of patients have carcinoid tumors

Symptoms independent from each other include cutaneous flushing, diarrhea, right cardiac valvular, and asthma

Common Curveballs

Carcinoid is less than 2 cm but invades appendiceal fat

Patient asks for other options besides right hemicolectomy for 1 cm carcinoid at appendiceal base

Patient has carcinoid syndrome with a carcinoid tumor you cannot locate

Patient presents with episodic flushing and diarrhea

Patient has liver metastases and may require lobectomy to fully debulk

Patient has ampullary carcinoid requiring a Whipple procedure to fully excise

Patient has an intraoperative carcinoid crisis

Patient presents with SBO secondary to tumor (path=small bowel carcinoid)

Examiner asks about the use of medication to treat carcinoid syndrome

Examiner asks about the indication for cholecystecomy

Clean Kills

Forgetting full physical examination (patient will have rectal carcinoid)

Forgetting adequate preoperative workup in patient with carcinoid syndrome (patient will have tricuspid or pulmonic valvular disease)

Forgetting the characteristics that determine the surgical treatment of carcinoid tumors

Failing to perform the appropriate cancer operation with resection of accompanying mesentery/lymph nodes

Failing to perform full exploratory laparotomy to rule out other carcinoid tumors in small bowel

Failing to recognize the carcinoid syndrome when present

Summary

Once you make the diagnosis of carcinoid, remember that size really does matter. In addition, location and extend of disease will drive extent of surgery. Review the

medical therapy to control symptoms, crisis, and recurrence. For emergent surgery, if your intraoperative level of suspicion is high for carcinoid, open exploration with pathology and a one-stage cancer operation is ideal.

Cushing's Syndrome

Concept

The majority of Cushing's syndrome cases are from an adrenocorticotropic hormone (ACTH)-secreting tumor of the pituitary gland. Other possible etiologies include an ectopic ACTH-producing tumor, adrenal adenoma, adrenal carcinoma, and bilateral adrenal hyperplasia. The treatment of choice is surgical resection.

Cushing Syndrome vs. Disease

– Syndrome=signs and symptoms of hypercortisolism, regardless of cause

– Disease=syndrome caused by pituitary adenoma (microadenoma)

Way Question May Be Asked?

"A 28-year-old woman is referred to your office for generalized weakness, new-onset diabetes, and hypertension. On physical examination, she is obese and has a buffalo hump and moon facies. What do you want to do?" It might be given that the patient is referred to you with the diagnosis of Cushing's syndrome. Examiners will not want to waste time in the history and physical stage, for the most part—but you still must know them just in case. Most examiners will want to get at your algorithm for managing the patient (this goes for most scenarios).

How to Answer?

History

Steroid use—most common cause

History of cancer (ACTH-producing tumor of lung)=ACTH dependent is most common (bronchial carcinoid or small cell lung cancer)

Diabetes

Hypertension

Generalized weakness

Physical Examination

Buffalo hump

Truncal obesity

Striae

Moon facies

Plethora
Osteopenia

Diagnostic Tests
24-h urine for cortisol (most cost-effective test if incidentaloma)—most sensitive and specific
Plasma cortisol level at 8 a.m. and 8 p.m. (check for loss of diurnal variation)
For the ACTH level, there are two possibilities (normal level is 10–100 pg/ml):
1. If elevated, the patient has a pituitary tumor or ectopic ACTH-producing tumor.
2. If low, the patient has adrenal pathology.
For the dexamethasone suppression test, there are two possibilities:
1. Low-dose overnight dexamethasone suppression test: If cortisol suppresses, know it is Cushing's disease (pituitary adenoma) was suppressed … if remains high
2. High-dose overnight dexamethasone suppression test: Measure serum ACTH if high have either ectopic ACTH producing tumor → continue onto if suppresses then have pituitary origin if does not suppress then ectopic

If you still cannot determine, perform a corticotropin-releasing hormone stimulation test. Pituitary adenoma will increase ACTH. If ectopic, there will be no change to ACTH.

Obtain magnetic resonance imaging (MRI) of the pituitary mass if suspected: remove transphenoidal approach and unresected pituitary tumors treated with XRT.

Next, obtain CT scans as follows:
Perform CT of the chest/abdomen/pelvis for an ectopic cancer source.
Perform CT of the abdomen for an adrenal source (can get thin-slice MRI adrenal).
  You should see the contralateral gland to be atrophied.
  You should not see bilateral enlargement.
  If >5 cm, suspect adrenocortical carcinoma.
Surgery
  Laparoscopic vs. open posterior unilateral adrenalectomy unless you suspect malignancy
  For adrenocortical carcinoma, resection includes adrenal, kidney, and continuous structures (spleen, distal pancreas, diaphragm).
  If metastatic disease is present, debulk.
  Medical treatment for ectopic ACTH production or adrenocortical cancer with residual metastasis is as follows:
Ketoconazole and metyrapone—inhibits steroid formation
Aminoglutethimide—inhibits cholesterol conversion
Op-DDD(miotane)—adrenal-lytic, used for metastatic disease only

Common Curveballs

Scenario changes with the first presentation as a pituitary tumor, then presentation as adrenal tumor
Tumor is malignant
Patient becomes Addisonian postoperatively
Examiner asks the difference between Cushing's syndrome and Cushing's disease
There is an ACTH- or corticotropin-releasing factor-secreting tumor (typically lung)
Patient is not a surgical candidate—treat medically as described above
You are given the results of tests you order (24-h urine cortisol, plasma cortisol levels, ACTH levels, dexamethasone suppression test)
Examiner asks when to order the above tests
– Case presents as an incidentaloma
– You need to figure out if functional or malignant
– Evaluate size (high-risk cancer if >6 cm)
– Get MRI/CT scans. Benign lesions will be smooth, round, and homogenous with low intensity on CT scan.
– Cancers of the adrenal are heterogeneous and may have calcifications.
– Most incidentalomas are nonfunctional.
– Removal all tumors greater than 4 cm (current recommendation).
– A patient with a nonfunctional tumor less than 4 cm should be followed with repeat CT scan at 3 months and 1 year.
Examiner asks to describe your surgical approach to adrenalectomy.

Clean Kills

Not being able to diagnose location of tumor
Not knowing treatment for pituitary tumor
Not knowing treatment for adrenal tumor
Performing fine needle aspiration (FNA) on the adrenal tumor: cytology from FNA cannot distinguish benign adrenal mass from carcinoma
Not recognizing the adrenal tumor for what it is and directing therapy towards a pituitary lesion

Summary

When a patient presents to the office with physical and hormonal changes leading you believe they might have a state of "hyper-cortisolism," it is very important to get a detailed history and a complete physical exam. The workup most commonly begins with laboratory values specific to determine where the cortisol is coming from.

Many of these tests are done by an endocrinologist in the office or in the hospital. Radiographic imaging is also an important modality for determining the locations of either a pituitary adenoma, adrenal pathology, or ectopic source of cortisol. Prior to any surgical intervention, a plan should be formulated in a multi-disciplinary team approach.

Hyperthyroidism

Concept

Hyperthyroidism has multiple etiologies, with surgical treatment reserved only for very specific indications. It is important to know how to make a diagnosis, the various treatment options, when to treat with surgery, and how to treat a hyperthyroid crisis.

Way Question May Be Asked?

"A 27-year-old woman is referred to your office by a family practitioner with the recent diagnosis of hyperthyroidism. What do you want to do?"

The patient may have symptoms of hyperthyroidism and you need to make the diagnosis first: tachycardia, heat intolerance, weight loss, fatigue, and palpitations.

How to Answer?

Always complete history and physical examination.
History
    Anxiety
    Tremulousness
    Weight loss
    Sweating
    Heat intolerance
    Palpitations
Physical Examination
    Neck nodules
    Exophthalmoses
Differential diagnosis
    Surgical treatment is considered for:
    Grave's disease (most common)
    Toxic multi-nodular goiter (Plummer's disease)
    Hyperfunctioning adenoma
    Amiodarone-associated thyrotoxicosis (AAT)

Medical Management
    Subacute thyroiditis
    Riedel's thyroiditis (invasive fibrous thyroiditis)

    Factitious thyrotoxicosis (exogenous T4)
    Ovarian (struma ovarii = thyroid tissue in ovarian teratoma), testicular, pituitary tumors (rarest)

Laboratory Tests
    Thyroid-stimulating hormone (TSH)
    Free T4
    Long-acting thyroid stimulant (LATS) level (Graves disease!)
    Thyroid antibody (thyroiditis)
    Thyroid scan (to rule out "hot" nodule)
    Ultrasound of the neck (to rule out mass)

Management
1. Medication (not for patients with toxic nodules)
    (a) Propylthyriouracil (PTU) or methimazole (Tapazole) is highly effective for Graves disease but not for toxic goiter. Problems include compliance and complications of medications, including agranulocytosis.
    (b) PTU can be used in pregnant patients.
2. Radioactive iodine (I^{131})
    (a) Good option in older patients
    (b) A single dose is usually effective in Graves disease and causse hypothyroidism in >90 %; has no role in AAT
    (c) Contraindicated in pregnant females, lactating mothers, and 1 year prior to pregnancy, so surgery is recommended for these cases
3. Glucocorticoid steroids
    (a) Rapidly lower T4 conversion to T3; however there are many side effects
4. Surgery
    (a) Lobectomy or subtotal thyroidectomy for toxic nodules
    (b) Subtotal thyroidectomy is appropriate for:
        Cosmesis
        Pregnant patients in the second trimester who fail PTU
        Failure of medical treatment after 1–2 years
        Compressive symptoms (goiters, riedels)
        Hyperthyroidism in children
        Young women who want to become pregnant
        Thyrocardiac patients
        Patients with severe exophthalmos
    (c) Need to prepare patient for surgery:
        PTU until surgery
        Beta blockers as needed (if used, continue in the postoperative period!)
        Lugol's solution (iodine) 2 cc twice daily starting 10–14 days prior to surgery to decrease vascularity of thyroid gland
        Continue beta blockers postoperatively for 8–10 days ($t_{1/2}$ of hormone)

(d) Thyroxin for life postoperatively (cannot tell true thyroid status until 1–2 years postoperatively)

Thyroid Storm

Thyroid storm is life-threatening!

It is initiated by physiologic stresses (surgery, anesthesia, myocardial infarction [MI], infection, childbirth).

Patients present with fever, tachycardia, abdominal symptoms, and change mental status.

Mortality is approximately 10 %.

Treatment for thyroid storm is as follows:

Intravenous fluid (IVF)

Sedatives

Oxygen; may need intubation

Antipyretics, cooling blankets

PTU 250 mg every 4 h

Hydrocortisone 100 every 6 h

Beta blockers (may need intravenous [IV] propranolol to control cardiac arrhythmias)

Lugol's solutions

Treat precipitating cause!

Common Curveballs

Patient has a hot nodule

Patient has a postoperative complication of

laryngeal nerve injury,

hematoma,

hypothyroidism,

injury to external branch of superior laryngeal nerve, or recurrent hyperthyroidism

Patient is pregnant

Patient fails medical therapy

Examiner asks to describe subtotal thyroidectomy (leave 3–5 g tissue behind)

Examiner asks how to prepare the patient prior to surgery

Patient has nodule that will be a malignancy on ultrasound, FNA, or final pathology (scenario switch)

Patient develops thyroid storm

Clean Kills

Not making the correct diagnosis

Not knowing how to treat hyperthyroidism

Not knowing indications for surgery

Not knowing how to treat/recognize thyroid storm

Not ruling out adenoma/malignancy

Not checking LATS, thyroid ultrasound, or T4/TSH

Not being comfortable with the discussion of complications of thyroidectomy

Summary

Surgical treatment for hyperthyroidism has clear indications and therefore could be an easy kill for you. Therefore, take your time and make the diagnosis. If the question involves a young woman, you must be able to counsel the patient about pregnancy treatment options. If hyperthyroidism is the topic, be prepared for thyroid storm because the forecast is rain.

Insulinoma

Concept

Insulinoma is a tumor in the pancreas that releases insulin. It is associated with multiple endocrine neoplasia (MEN) type 1 syndrome (pituitary, pancreas, parathyroid), so be sure to ask about family history. The tumor is usually less than 2 cm in size; if it is >3 cm, be suspicious of malignancy. Management depends on tumor location, number of tumors, malignancy, and whether it is a part of MEN syndrome (hyperparathyroidism, pituitary/pancreatic tumors). You need to rule out other causes for hypoglycemia, such as liver disorder (cirrhosis, Gaucher's disease), pregnancy, and exogenous administration. This is the most common functional tumor of the endocrine pancreas (for those tumors not in the MEN syndromes, gastrinoma is the most common).

Way Question May Be Asked?

"A 37-year-old woman presents with a history of repeated bouts of weakness and fatigue after meals, with a fasting glucose level of 40."

There are several ways the question can go. However, after ruling out liver disorder and alcoholism, (quickly) start focusing on insulinoma. Rarely will you be presented with the classic Whipple's triad of

symptoms with fasting,

blood glucose < 50 at time of symptoms, and

symptoms that are relieved with glucose administration.

How to Answer?

You will need to perform a complete history and physical examination.

History

Syncope

Blurred vision

Sweating that is brought on by fasting or exercise

Palpitations

Weakness

Seizures

Confusion

Family history of MENI syndrome

Early pregnancy could be mistaken for this syndrome.

Diagnostic Studies

Diagnosis usually made during a 72-h fast.

You need to monitor the fasting test to prevent life-threatening hypoglycemia and to rule out factitious hypoglycemia from exogenous administration.

You need to have a <u>fasting glucose</u> level (should be less than 60).

You need to check <u>fasting insulin</u> level (should be greater than 24).

Check <u>insulin-to-glucose</u> ratio (should be >0.3).

Check <u>C-terminal peptide</u> level to rule out exogenous insulin administration (will *not* be elevated only with exogenous insulin; a level higher than 1.2 with a glucose level less than 40 is highly suggestive of insulinoma).

You could also check <u>proinsulin</u> level (elevated with insulinoma).

You will need to try to localize insulinoma (80 % in pancreas, may be multiple if familial variety, only 10 % malignant).

There is equal distribution in the head, body, and tail (97 %).

The remaining 3 % may be in the duodenum, splenic hilum, or gastrocolic ligament.

Localization Studies Do not stop after the CT scan!

1. CT scan of abdomen and pelvis with thin cuts through pancreas—sensitivity is directly related to size of the tumor. This tumor is smaller so it is more difficult to localize.
2. Arteriogram—will detect 70 % of insulinomas larger than 5 mm, showing a characteristic vascular blush
3. Portosplenic vein sampling (be prepared for results of this test!)—can stimulate with calcium because it will stimulate insulin release from the tumor
4. Endoscopic ultrasound—93 % overall sensitivity for tumors of any size
5. MRI

Even if you cannot localize the tumor (and you usually will not be able to), you can start the patient on diazoxide and prepare the patient for surgery (be sure the patient is an acceptable surgical candidate).

Surgical Treatment

In the operating room (OR), you need to fully examine the pancreas by division of the gastrohepatic ligament, Kocher maneuver, medial reflection of spleen, and division of the peritoneum on the superior and inferior borders of the pancreas.

The entire abdomen must be explored, with particular attention paid to possible liver metastasis.

If performing an enucleation, administer a dose of secretin intraoperatively to check for leaks, place the omental flap, and leave a drain.

Then, you will be in one of the following situations:

1. You find a tumor in the head of pancreas: Perform enucleation (may get pancreatic fistula postoperatively)
   - You should not perform enucleation if the mass is within 2 mm of the main pancreatic duct distal to the pancreas; instead perform distal pancreatectomy
   - The procedure can be performed laparoscopically.
2. You find a tumor in the pancreas with metastasis: Perform debulking surgery and use somatostatin, diazoxide, and streptozotocin postoperatively.
   - You can perform hepatic artery embolization.
3. You cannot find a tumor: Perform intraoperative ultrasound and rapid venous assays
   (a) If you still cannot find the tumor, try to send to outside facility for rapid venous assays to detect drop in insulin level.
   (b) If examiner will not let you do that, perform a distal pancreatectomy and send for frozen section and glucose/insulin measurement.
   (c) Do not perform a near total pancreatectomy unless you are an endocrine expert.
4. MENI: Perform a subtotal pancreatectomy because of the high incidence of islet cell hyperplasia.

Patient may have mild hyperglycemia for 2–3 days postoperatively.

Common Curveballs

You are not able to localize tumor preoperatively

You are not able to localize tumor intraoperatively (consider intraoperative ultrasound)

You do not have facilities to do rapid venous sampling

You find a mass and FNA shows a malignant adenocarcinoma

Patient has multiple tumors

Patient has pancreatic duct leak after enucleation

There is exogenous administration if you did not check C-terminal peptide/proinsulin level

Patient has MEN syndrome

Patient has malignant tumor

You cannot enucleate because of deep tumor in head/tail of pancreas (if you do, there will be damage to pancreatic duct)

You perform distal pancreatectomy, patient is still symptomatic, and the examiner asks if you regret your decision

(stick to your guns if you know you gave the right answer—the examiner is most likely trying to determine how confident a surgeon you are)

Will be pancreatic duct leak after enucleation

Clean Kills

Whipple procedure for tumor near surface (appropriate if deep in pancreatic head)

Stopping after CT scan and proceeding straight to OR

Failing to ask about family history that is suspicious for MEN (pituitary, pancreas, parathyroid problems)

Failing to rule out exogenous insulin administration

Performing too radical a surgery before an exhaustive workup, including venous sampling and possible referral to a center specializing in the disease (always better to refer the patient to a tertiary care center than blindly performing a near total pancreatectomy)

Not mentioning controlling symptoms preoperatively with small, frequent meals or diazoxide (suppresses insulin secretion, with side effects of fluid retention and nausea)

Failing to rule out liver disease

Failing to recognize insulin-producing tumor in a patient with hypoglycemic symptoms reversible with sugar intake

Not knowing the Whipple's triad

Performing a pancreatic resection when you identified a tumor near the surface rather than enucleation

Describing the exploration and enucleation to be done laparoscopically

Mistaking the surgery for gastrinoma for insulinoma, opening up the duodenum and palpating for tumor

It is always okay to say, "I don't perform this procedure, but the key steps are…" This answer is better than describing a procedure you do not perform, then being backed up against the wall when asked questions about technical steps in the procedure.

Summary

Although insulinoma is the most common functional endocrine tumor, the chance of seeing patient with an insulinoma is still rare. The common presentation includes hypoglycemia during fasting, which resolves with glucose administration. Most importantly, it is crucial to determine whether this is true oversecretion of insulin or exogenous administration as seen in Munchausen syndrome. History, including a family history, could identify risk factors of MEN syndrome. Laboratory studies, including secretin stimulation testing, is important in making the diagnosis. After the diagnosis

is confirmed, imaging studies are used to localize the tumor. Surgical resection is facilitated if localization is successful; if not, full inspection of the pancreas should always be completed. Intraoperative ultrasound and venous sampling are sometimes used.

Pheochromocytoma

Concept

Pheochromocytoma is a tumor of the adrenal medulla that produces excess catecholamines. It originates from the chromaffin cells of the adrenal medulla in 90 % of cases. Approximately 10 % of cases are extra-adrenal, pediatric, malignant, bilateral, or familial (MENIIa or IIb). Other locations include sympathetic ganglia in the neck, abdomen, pelvis, mediastinum, and the organs of Zuckerandl.

- It is found more commonly in people with MENII, von Recklinghausen's neurofibromatosis, and von Hippel-Lindau disease.

Way Question May Be Asked?

"A 24-year-old woman is sent to you for evaluation of her frequent headaches, palpitations, and blood pressure of 190/110. What do you want to do?"

You may be given a history including flushing, sweating, episodic attacks, or a young patient with new-onset hypertension.

How to Answer?

History—secondary to excess catecholamines
    Frequent "attacks"
    Anxiety
    Sweating/flushing
    Headaches
    Hypertension (50 % sustained)
    Palpitations
    Family history (MENIIa—hyperparathyroid, pheochromocytoma, medullary thyroid cancer)
    Other neuroectodermal diseases (von Hippel-Lindau, tuberous sclerosis, neurofibromatosis)
    Predominate on the right side

Physical Examination
    Blood pressure
    Gentle abdominal examination (you do not want to compress the organ of Zuckerkandl)
    Palpate thyroid

Diagnostic Testing
> 24-h urine for vanillylmandelic acid (VMA), meta-nephrine, normetanephrine (make sure the patient is not on an monoamine oxidase inhibitor)—this is the criterion standard for disease, with 90 % sensitivity
>
> Ca^{++} and calcitonin levels (to rule out MENIIa)
>
> Can have false elevation in VMA with coffee, tea, fruits, vanilla, iodine, and labetalol
>
> Clonidine suppression test: tumor will not respond to treatment

Localization Studies
1. CT scan of the abdomen/pelvis
   Look at adrenals
   Look for extra-adrenal tumors
   Look for metastases
2. I-131 metaiodobenzylguanidine scan: accumulates in chromaffin tissue more rapidly in pheochromocytomas
3. Portosplenic vein sampling (be prepared for results of this test or to describe how it is performed!)
4. MRI
5. Do not perform venography; it will cause a hypertensive crisis

Surgical Treatment

You need to adequately prepare the patient pre-operatively.
1. Start an alpha blocker 2 weeks prior to surgery: phenoxy-benzamine 20 mg twice daily and increase by 20 mg/day until blood pressure and symptoms are controlled. The goal of this is to prevent an intra-operative hypertensive crisis.
2. Add beta blockers 3 days prior to surgery: propranolol 10 mg three times daily to lower heart rate
3. Start IVF hydration 2 days prior to surgery (these patients are volume contracted) to prevent circulatory collapse
   In the OR, have rapid-acting agents ready:
Neosynephrine
Lidocaine
Propranolol
Phentolamine (alpha-blocker)

Have a central venous pressure line (or swann ganz cathether (SGC)) and arterial line

Do not use MSO_4/Demerol (catechol release) or atropine (increases tachycardia)

Be prepared to describe right and left adrenalectomy and anatomy of adrenal vein on both sides!

Surgery

Make a midline incision: the open anterior approach is classic and allows for complete abdominal exploration

Perform full exploration of both adrenal glands, aortic bifurcation, bladder, kidney hilum

Control venous drainage first: ligate adrenal vein first to prevent spilling of catecholamines during tumor manipulation

Excise tumor with minimal manipulation

Debulk malignant tumors to help reduce symptoms

Bilateral adrenalectomy for bilateral disease, MENII

If you cannot locate the tumor, other possible sites include the vertebral body, the opposite adrenal gland, the bladder, and aortic bifurcation (the most common extra-adrenal site is the organ of Zuckerandl)

After the tumor is resected, give 1 mg of glucagon to check for occult tumors (tachycardia or increased blood pressure are signs of a residual tumor).

After resection, the patient may have hypertension, hypotension, hypoglycemia, bronchospasm, arrhythmias, cerebral hemorrhage, or MI.

Medical Treatment

Metyrosine: inhibits tyrosine hydroxylase, which causes decrease in synthesis of catecholamines

Follow-up

Urinary studies every 3 months, then yearly

Screen all family members yearly for pheochromocytoma, medullary thyroid cancer, and hyperparathyroidism

Common Curveballs

You are not able to localize preoperatively (still proceed with exploration in open fashion)

You are not able to localize intraoperatively (consider intra-operative ultrasound)

You do not have facilities to perform rapid venous sampling

Patient has multiple tumors

Patient has a malignant tumor

Patient has recurrent symptoms postoperatively (consider that you did not get all of the tumor)

Patient has MENII syndrome (which operation is performed first? Pheochromocytoma should be corrected first, then the medullary thyroid cancer)

Patient has intraoperative fluctuations of blood pressure and heart rate

Clean Kills

Failing to ask about family history

Not knowing preoperative workup or preoperative preparation of patient

Describing laparoscopic operation in a patient with evidence of metastases, prior operations, or large tumor (>8 cm)

Not ligating adrenal vein early in your description of operation

Not placing invasive hemodynamic devices intraoperatively

Not screening relatives (for RET proto-oncogene) if you suspect MENII syndrome

Summary

Pheochromocytoma is a tumor of the adrenal medulla commonly seen in MENII syndrome. Patients present with classic symptoms of episodic hypertension, diaphoresis, and anxiety. Urine metanephrines is the most sensitive and specific test to rule in pheochromocytoma. Multiple imaging modalities have been used to localize the phenol. The treatment of choice is surgical, but if the patient is not a surgical candidate medical palliation is also acceptable.

Primary Aldosteronism

Concept

Primary aldosteronism is either unilateral adenoma (85 %) or bilateral adrenal hyperplasia (15 %) resulting in elevated aldosterone levels, hypertension, and hypokalemia.

Way Question May Be Asked?

"A 32-year-old woman has a 2-year history of hypertension that is unresponsive to medical treatment."

The patient may also have fatigue, muscle cramps, polyuria, weight gain, and peripheral edema (often the first thing a patient notices is that rings do not fit on the fingers).

How to Answer?

You have to think about surgically correctable forms of hypertension in a young patient with new-onset hypertension (coarctation, renal artery stenosis, Cushing's disease, pheochromocytoma)

Complete history

    Questions to rule out pheochromocytoma

    Family history (if suspicious of pheochromocytoma)

    Make sure the patient is not taking any medications (especially diuretics, which will throw off laboratory values)

Complete physical examination

Check for low potassium on basic metabolic panel

Check aldosterone/renin ratio (should be >20 or primary hyperaldosteronism)

    If renin is high, suspect other etiology (renal artery stenosis, secondary disease)

To differentiate bilateral hyperplasia from adenoma, use the captopril test:

1. Give a dose of captopril and measure aldosterone levels before and after; if it decreases, then the patient has bilateral hyperplasia
2. Urine aldosterone after salt load is the best test—it will stay high
3. Decreased serum potassium, increased serum sodium, and metabolic alkalosis

Always try to localize tumor (these are typically small):

1. CT scan of the abdomen/pelvis
2. Selective venous sampling (especially if CT is negative)
3. NP-59 iodocholesterol scan (helps to rule out hyperplasia too)—will show hyperfunctioning adrenal tissue

If the diagnosis is bilateral hyperplasia, the treatment is medical with Spironolactone (effective in 90 % of cases; on the boards, it is unlikely to be this option)

If the diagnosis is single adenoma, unilateral adrenalectomy is indicated. This could be performed as follows:

1. A posterior approach through the 12th rib on the right or 11th rib on the left
2. Through a midline laparotomy
3. Laparoscopically

Describe whatever approach you are comfortable with, but remember the following:

1. On the right side, the adrenal vein enters posteriorly into the inferior vena cava (IVC) and mobilization of the right lobe of the liver is necessary if going transabdominal.
2. On the left side, mobilization of the colon and pancreas ± spleen may be required and the adrenal vein empties into the renal vein.
3. Only the venous drainage is consistent in adrenal anatomy.

Be careful of postoperative hypotension. You may need to use steroids.

Common Curveballs

Patient has hyperplasia if you haven't ruled it out

Patient has no tumor on CT scan, so know the other localizing studies

Patient has RAS or fibromuscular dysplasia if you haven't checked renin levels

Patient has postoperative hypotension (from adrenal insufficiency)

Spleen is injured when mobilizing colon for left adrenalectomy

IVC is injured during right adrenalectomy

Clean Kills

Not checking potassium, aldosterone, or renin levels

Not being able to describe the surgical approach (no matter what the question, this brings you back next year—and if you cannot describe it, do not make it up!)

Not ruling out other forms of surgically correctable hypertension

Not knowing medical treatment for bilateral hyperplasia and performing bilateral adrenalectomies

Not knowing how to treat postoperative hypotension and doing extensive workup for hemorrhagic/hypovolemic/cardiogenic shock

Misdiagnosing patient as having a pheochromocytoma

Not knowing the mechanism of action of aldosterone or the renin–angiotensin–aldosterone axis

Not knowing that the syndrome is nicknamed Conn's syndrome

Summary

Hyperaldosteronism (also known as Conn's syndrome) typically presents with hypertension and hypokalemia. Basic laboratory studies should be ordered. Because these tumors are typically small, localization with preoperative imaging is key. If unilateral, adrenalectomy is indicated. Bilateral disease is usually treated with medical treatment.

Head and Neck Endocrine

Anna Goldenberg Sandau and Roy L. Sandau

Neck Mass

Concept

Neck masses are usually benign. (However, a neck mass will not be benign during the boards!) Differential diagnosis should be complete, and your history and physical examination should guide you towards the underlying process. Follow the rule of 80s after age 40:

80 % of nonthyroid neck masses in adults are neoplastic

80 % of neoplastic masses are malignant

80 % of malignant masses are metastatic

80 % of malignancies in adults are squamous cell carcinomas

80 % of metastases are from primary sites above the level of the clavicle

Be wary of a neck mass in an infant, in the midline, or in a patient with human immunodeficiency virus (HIV) (lymphoma).

Way Question May Be Asked?

"A 43-year-old man presents to the office with a mass in his left neck. It is non-tender and has been there for about 3 months. He has a significant smoking history. What do you want to do?"

How to Answer?

History
   Age (very important here)
   Location (again, very important)
   Duration
   Drainage (branchial cyst?)
   Pain
   Tobacco/alcohol use
   Hoarseness
   Dysphagia
   History (HIV+, prior malignancy)
   Systemic symptoms ("B symptoms" with lymphoma?)
   Previous head/neck surgery (Was a suspicious mole/melanoma removed? Was it overlying the parotid gland?)
Physical Examination
   Location
   Tenderness
   Fixed/mobile
   Movement with swallowing
   Pulsatile (the rare carotid body tumor)
   Sinus (branchial cyst)
   Nasopharynx
   Oral cavity
   Larynx
   Neck (thyroid)
   Other lymph node basins (axillary, groin)
   Skin
   Breast
   Abdomen (palpable liver/spleen)
   Stool guitar (maybe metastatic)
Diagnostic Tests
   Fine needle aspiration (FNA; critical here and helpful in neck masses!)
   Chest x-ray (CXR; lung or mediastinal pathology)
   Computed tomography (CT) scan of the face/neck (sinuses/oral cavity/nasopharynx/larynx)
   ± Magnetic resonance imaging (MRI)
   ± Ultrasound of neck (useful to evaluate thyroid/parathyroid)
   ± Thyroid scan (again, useful to evaluate thyroid/parathyroid)
   Blood tests (as always, complete laboratory panels and complete blood count with differential; in select cases, include calcitonin/calcium levels, thyroid hormones, and examination of blood smear)

A.G. Sandau, D.O. (✉)
General Surgery, University of Medicine and Dentistry of New Jersey, School of Osteopathic Medicine, Stratford, NJ, USA
e-mail: agolde5044@yahoo.com

R.L. Sandau, D.O.
General Surgery, Kennedy University Hospital, 2201 Chapel Ave West, Suite 100, Cherry Hill, NJ 08002, USA

M.A. Neff (ed.), *Passing the General Surgery Oral Board Exam*,
DOI 10.1007/978-1-4614-7663-4_5, © Springer Science+Business Media New York 2014

Differential Diagnosis
  Midline
    Thyroglossal duct cyst
    Dermoid cysts
    Pyramidal lobe of thyroid

  Lateral
    Lymph node—infected vs. metastatic
    Brachial cleft cyst

  Supraclavicular
    Lymph node—infected vs. metastatic

  Submandibular/Pre-auricular mass
    Lymph node
    Parotid gland
    Salivary gland
  Do not forget inflammatory etiologies of enlarged lymph nodes:
  Lymphadenitis
  Tuberculosis
  Tularemia
  Cat scratch
  Toxoplasmosis
  Sarcoidosis
  Viral

Treatment

Thyroglossal duct cyst
  Ultrasound of the neck to confirm presence of normal thyroid
  Excision with middle portion of hyoid bone; follow any tissue to base of tongue (Sistrunk procedure)
Brachial cleft cyst (always surgical excision, be careful of the anatomic pathway!)
  First brachial cleft:
    Opening at angle of mandible, passes through facial nerve
  Second brachial cleft (most common):
    Opening anterior border of the sternocleidomastoid muscle (SCM), passes between carotid bifurcation
  Third brachial cleft:
    Opening at lower border of SCM, passes behind carotid

Lymph node = squamous cell carcinoma
Nasopharyngeal laryngoscopy (in your office)
Excisional biopsy under anesthesia plus examination under anesthesia with the following:

Panendoscopy of upper aerodigestive tract
  Direct laryngoscopy
  Rigid esophagoscopy
  Rigid bronchoscopy
Biopsies of nasopharynx, base of tongue, pyriform sinus
Excision of primary site (if found) and modified radical neck dissection

Lymph node = adenocarcinoma
CT scan of neck/chest/abdomen/pelvis
Bilateral mammograms
Esophagogastroduodenoscopy
Barium Enema (BE)/colonoscopy
If primary is found, this represents stage 4 disease and chemotherapy may be offered.
If no primary is found, perform excisional biopsy plus modified radical neck dissection on that side.
Send for ER/PR receptors and mucin stain (to rule out melanoma/lymphoma)

Lymph node = thyroid
Thyroid ultrasound
Thyroid scan
Total thyroidectomy
  Enlarged nodes for papillary cancer
  Central lymph node dissection and modified radical neck dissection for medullary

Lymph node = lymphoma
Excisional biopsy of node
CT scan of the neck/chest/abdomen/pelvis
Bone marrow biopsy (stage IV disease)
Stage disease (number of nodal groups/which side of diaphragm)
Staging laparotomy?
Chemotherapy (cyclophosphamide-hydroxydaunorubicin-Oncovin-prednisone [CHOP])
  Postoperative radiotherapy to neck should be considered after radical neck dissection
  Important anatomy to remember:

Anterior triangle boundaries
Lateral = SCM
Medial = midline of neck
Superior = inferior edge of mandible

Posterior triangle boundaries
Inferior = clavicle
Anterior = SCM
Posterior = trapezius

Steps in radical neck dissection

T-incision

Locate and protect mandibular and cervical branches of facial nerves

Divide anterior facial vessels

Remove contents of submental and submandibular triangles

Ligate external jugular vein close to subclavian

Protect spinal accessory, phrenic, and brachial plexus while removing fat/lymphatic tissue in posterior triangle

Low division of omohyoid behind SCM

Division of SCM

Open carotid sheath and ligate Internal Jugular (IJ) close to clavicle

Ligate submaxillary duct

In modified radical neck dissection, the following are preserved:

Spinal accessory nerve

Internal jugular vein

SCM

Common Curveballs

Patient has metastatic thyroid cancer

FNA is indeterminate

Scenario switches several times from squamous cell carcinoma to adenocarcinoma to lymphoma

Melanoma overlies the parotid gland (modified radical neck plus superficial parotidectomy)

You are not able to identify the primary site

You find the primary site and are asked how to perform resection

Patient has seroma under the skin flap

Patient has chylous fistula in left neck dissection

Patient has carotid blowout postoperatively

Patient has damage to a nerve (phrenic, spinal accessory, vagus, hypoglossal)

Clean Kills

Not knowing the different algorithms between FNA yielding squamous cell carcinoma vs. lymphoma vs. adenocarcinoma

Not having a broad differential diagnosis

Not performing FNA

Not knowing the surgical procedure for
thyroglossal duct cyst or the
most common branchial cleft cyst

Not being able to describe modified neck dissection or the difference from a complete radical dissection

Summary

This topic is really a test of how well you can develop a differential diagnosis and to "rule things out" through your workup. Therefore, you will likely have to ask some more questions on your history and physical examination regardless of the way the scenario is given to you. Look for clues as to where the mass is (may be given "left anterior neck") and the age/sex of the patient to help guide you. A wide battery of laboratory and diagnostic tests will help to make the diagnosis for you. From here, it should be all downhill.

Hyperparathyroidism

Concept

Hyperparathyroidism is one of many possible causes of hypercalcemia. You must rule out common causes of hypercalcemia first, then remember the primary, secondary, and tertiary types of hyperparathyroidism:

1. Primary hyperparathyroidism: ~80 % adenoma and ~2 % double adenoma
2. Secondary hyperparathyroidism from hyperplasia is often secondary to renal failure
3. Tertiary hyperparathyroidism is from autonomous functioning glands after the etiology causing the secondary hyperparathyroidism has been treated (most common in renal transplant patients)

Way Question May Be Asked?

"A 61-year-old woman has an elevated calcium level on routine blood tests. Her only complaint is fatigue. What do you want to do?"

"A 72-year-old woman has fatigue and constipation."

Sometimes you will be given symptoms of renal stones, abdominal pain, constipation, arthralgia, myalgia, depression, ulcers, pancreatitis, osteitis fibrosa cystica, but rarely all of the symptoms associated with elevated calcium (renal stones, bone pain, constipation, fatigue, ulcer, depression, emotional lability, etc.).

How to Answer?

First, you need to be able to rule out common causes of hypercalcemia. Many mnemonics can be used here, but all include vitamin D deficiency, malignancy (breast, lung, prostate, multiple myeloma), primary and secondary hyperparathyroidism, sarcoidosis, thiazides, immobilization, familial hypocalciuric hypercalcemia, milk-alkali syndrome, and hyperthyroidism.

Second, to document hyperparathyroidism, you need to confirm hypercalcemia on repeat blood tests. Other laboratory tests are needed to confirm.

1. Rule out vitamin D deficiency and check vitamin 25-OH D levels
2. Check Cl/PO_4 level (greater than 30 is suggestive of primary hyperparathyroidism)
3. Get parathyroid hormone (PTH) level
4. Low PO_4 (high in renal failure)
5. Serum albumin to correct for serum calcium or ionized calcium
6. 24-h urinary calcium for rare hypercalcemic hypocalciuria

Indications for Asymptomatic Patients

1. Serum calcium 1.0 mg/dL than normal
2. 24-h urine is no longer indicated
3. Creatine clearance <60 mL/min
4. Bone mineral density—2.5 z-score at any site (distal one-third radius is preferred)
5. ± previous fracture fragility

Localization (in order)

1. Ultrasound: Determine 2 mm of detail and identify thyroid nodules that may need workup prior to parathyroid surgery.
2. Sestamibi scan: 80 % are positive; however, if negative, the patient is still most likely to have a single adenoma.
3. CT or MRI are performed only when ultrasound and sestamibi scan are negative.
4. If all tests are negative, surgical exploration is indicated.
5. Venous sampling is reserved for failed exploration.

Procedure

Adenoma

1. If sestamibi is positive, excise adenoma using intraoperative gamma probe; you can offer local mini-incision (<2 cm)
2. If tumor is not localized preoperatively, you must identify all four glands prior to excision.
3. If the intraoperative PTH level is available, wait 10–15 min; a 50 % drop from the preoperative level is confirmatory.

4. Frozen sections can be done; the pathologist should confirm adenoma and enlarged gland by weight.
5. If the intraoperative PTH level is not available, you must biopsy all glands for frozen section. Reimplant if a 3.5 excision is done.

Hyperplasia

1. Take all four glands and autotransplant into the nondominant forearm.
2. If the intraoperative PTH level is available, you should draw after all four glands are removed to test for a fifth gland.
3. Offer cryopreservation of the gland.

Cancer

1. The PTH level typically is >1,000. Perform en bloc resection of the parathyroid gland, ipsilateral lymph nodes, and thyroid lobectomy.
   #### If you cannot find a gland
1. If it is an upper gland, check the paraesophageal and retrolaryngeal spaces as well as the posterior mediastinum. Perform a thyroid lobectomy on that side.
2. If it is a lower gland, check the tracheoesophageal groove, carotid sheath, thymus, thyroid, and anterior mediastinum.
3. If you still cannot find a gland, do not perform a sternotomy the first time around. Follow postoperative Ca/PTH levels.

Common Curveballs

Patient postoperatively has persistently elevated calcium/or comes back in 6 months with elevated calcium. In this case, be methodical with a complete workup including calcium, phosphorus, and PTH levels; MRI, sestamibi, and ultrasound. This is one of four situations:

1. Missed adenoma (most likely)—could be a fifth gland in the mediastinum or on the same side
2. Missed hyperplasia
3. Parathyroid carcinoma
4. Parathyromosis

You are not able to find four glands

Patient has more than four glands

Examiner asks when you would consider cryopreservation of any of the glands

Condition is part of a multiple endocrine neoplasia (MEN) syndrome

Patient has postoperative hypocalcemia

Patient has postoperative airway compromise

Patient has postoperative hoarseness

Patient is sent to you after previously failed neck exploration elsewhere

Examiner asks you to comment on why four-gland exploration is better than exploration on just one side (to justify whatever position you offer)

Patient presents very subtly with only fatigue or renal stones

Examiner asks innocent questions, such as "How does PTH work?"(increases bone resorption, increases renal resorption of Ca and renal secretion of phos, and stimulates vitamin D formation)

Examiner asks how to manage a hypercalcemic crisis (treat with IVF, Lasix, steroids, calcitonin, surgery when stable)

Patient has parathyroid carcinoma

Patient has postoperative hematoma

Patient has negative sestamibi scan (see above)

Examiner asks what to do if intraoperative PTH level increases after excision of adenoma (double adenoma and explore)

Examiner asks about medications Sensipar (cinacalcet) and Rocaltrol (calcitriol)

Examiner asks about methylene blue injection during procedure (only mention if they keep on questioning what else can you do)

Clean Kills

Failing to rule out MEN syndrome

Failing to rule out common causes of hypercalcemia

Performing median sternotomy first time around when you find only three glands

Finding a single adenoma and stopping operation

Not knowing how to deal with postoperative persistent hypercalcemia

Not knowing how PTH works

Not knowing the indications for surgery

Not knowing the percentage for finding a single adenoma (80 %)

Not knowing how to deal with postoperative complications

Not knowing where to look for the "missing" upper or lower gland

Summary

Parathyroid surgery for hyperparathyroidism could be a very difficult question with a vague presentation. A very careful history and workup will keep you on the right track. Preoperative laboratory tests and localization should be exhausted to show you are operating for the right diagnosis. Intraoperative localization techniques, anatomy, and confirmation methods will always be asked. Know what to do after surgery if you cannot not find the gland or the patient experiences hypocalcemia or nerve injury. You cannot go wrong if you transfer the patient to a high-volume center for reoperative surgery.

Thyroid Nodule

Concept

A thyroid nodule may be a "hot" nodule, benign adenoma, malignancy, or other neck mass (parathyroid, lymph node).

Way Question May Be Asked?

"A 31-year-old woman was seen by her primary care physician recently for a sore throat. She was noted to have a mass on the left side of her thyroid. What do you want to do?"

You may be presented with a mass found by a family medicine physician and sent to you or you may be given symptoms of hyperthyroidism. After your initial history and physical examination, all patients should get ultrasound and FNA.

How to Answer?

History
  Questions related to hyper- or hypothyroidism
    Tachycardia
    Heat intolerance
    Weight loss/gain
    Fatigue
    Depression
    Cold intolerance
    History of radiation to neck (breast cancer/Hodgkin's disease)
    History of new hoarseness/changes in voice
    Any possibility of MEN syndrome (ask about pheochromocytoma and hypercalcemia—about 10 % of medullary thyroid cancers are associated with MEN)
    Family history: goiter, MENII, thyroid cancer
    Diarrhea (medullary)

Physical Examination
  Attention to description of the mass
  Cervical lymph nodes
  Examination of vocal cords if new-onset hoarseness
  Reflexes, pulse, blood pressure (hyperthyroidism)
  Fixed vs. mobile, movement with deglutition

Diagnostic Tests
  FNA—simple to perform in office setting

Ultrasound—helps look for other nodules, determine solid vs. cystic

Thyroid scan (cold vs. hot nodule)

Blood tests: T4, TSH, thyroglobulin level (for follow-up), thyroid antibodies, calcitonin and Ca++ level (if you suspect medullary cancer).

Be ready for Ca++ to be elevated and for a scenario switch!

If you suspect pheochromocytoma, get calcitonin, serum calcium, phosphate, and urine studies for pheochromocytoma, as well as RET testing

Results of FNA

1. Insufficient sample: Repeat FNA
2. Benign: Repeat ultrasound and physical examination in 6–12 months
3. Malignant: surgery
4. Indeterminate:
   (a) Follicular cells/Hurthle cells: 15–25 % malignant.
       - If patient is <45 years of age and if nodule is ≤2 cm, then observation and lobectomy is appropriate.
       - If patient is >45 of age or neoplasm ≥2 cm and patient history indicates high risk, then perform a total thyroidectomy.
   (b) Suspicious: 50–75 % malignant.
       - If patient is <45 years of age and if nodule is ≤1 cm, then observation and lobectomy are appropriate. For bilateral nodules, perform a total thyroidectomy.
       - If patient is >45 years of page or neoplasm is ≥1 cm and patient history indicates high risk, then perform a total thyroidectomy.

Surgical Treatment

1. Lobectomy
   (a) Papillary cancer less than 1 cm (microcarcinoma)
2. Total thyroidectomy
   (a) Follicular cancer
   (b) Bilateral multinodular micropapillary
3. Total thyroidectomy with central neck dissection
   (a) Papillary cancer >1 cm
   (b) Medullary cancer
   (c) Hurthle cell cancer
4. Total thyroidectomy with modified radical lymph node dissection (sparing the sternocleidomastoid muscle and spinal accessory nerve)
   (a) Any well-differentiated cancer with the presence of clinically palpable or ultrasound-positive lateral to carotid sheath lymph nodes
5. Total thyroidectomy, en bloc resection, modified radical lymph node dissection, ± tracheostomy, ± chemoradiation therapy

(a) Anaplastic cancer

Postoperative Cancer Treatment

Postoperative treatment may include replacement hormones, withdrawal, thyroid scan, I^{131} ablation, and TSH suppression as low as the patient can tolerate.

Options

1. Synthroid (levothyroxine), then a low-iodine diet and withdrawal ×4 weeks prior to ablation
2. Cytomel (liothyronine), low-iodine diet, and withdrawal ×2 weeks prior to ablation
3. Synthroid, no withdrawal, but thyrogen (thyrotropin, recombinant TSH) injections ×2 days then ablation on the third day

Surveillance

1. Thyroglobulin levels, anti-thryoglobulin antibody levels (calcitonin for medullary cancer)
2. Yearly ultrasounds
3. Radioiodine scan every 6 months

Common Curveballs

Patient has postoperative airway compromise

Patient has postoperative vocal cord paralysis

Examiner asks about possible nerve injuries (recurrent laryngeal and superior laryngeal) and their consequences

Patient has postoperative hypocalcemia

Condition is part of a MEN syndrome

Patient has follicular cells on FNA

Examiner ask you to justify your reasoning for total thyroidectomy

Patient has nodules in both lobes

Patient has a goiter plus a nodule

Patient has thyroglobulin levels that increase several months postoperatively

Thyroid scan shows a "hot nodule"

Clean Kills

Failing to rule out MEN syndrome

Not knowing how to deal with postoperative complications

Not performing an FNA

Not knowing when to follow calcitonin levels (medullary carcinoma) and when to follow thyroglobulin levels

Not performing central node dissection in medullary carcinoma

Not placing the patient on postoperative thyroxin

Summary

The thyroid nodule workup always starts with an ultrasound-guided FNA. The key is what do you do from there. You have to be able to extensively defend your surgical options for lobectomy versus total thyroidectomy. Postoperative management of complications and cancer follow-up is always a guaranteed question. If tests lead to medullary cancer, be prepared for a MEN syndrome workup.

Esophagus

Christina Sanders

Zenker's Diverticulum

Concept

In Zenker's diverticulum, upper esophageal muscle dyscoordination occurs with the lower pharyngeal constrictor contracting against an unyielding cricopharyngeus muscle. This condition causes an acquired (false diverticulum) mucosal outpouching of the esophageal wall between these muscles on the left posterolateral side. (Killian's triangle).

Way Question May Be Asked?

"A 78-year-old man presents on referral from his family doctor complaining of trouble swallowing with occasional regurgitation of undigested food, mainly at night."

Rarely will you be presented with a patient with obvious bad breath, dysphagia to solids and liquids, regurgitation of undigested food, a sensation of a lump in the throat, and gurgling in the neck. Weight loss and aspiration are late symptoms.

How to Answer?

You must work through an algorithm of dysphagia and rule out achalasia and cancer.

Full History
- Dysphagia to solids versus liquids
- Weight loss
- Smoking
- Gastroesophageal reflux disease (GERD)/Barrett's esophagus

Coughing up solid food
Halitosis (bad breath)
Gurgling in neck
Sensation of something stuck in throat
Recurrent respiratory infections
Voice changes
Excessive salivation
Substernal chest pain

Full Physical Examination
- Neck and lymph node basins (will never feel diverticulum)

Diagnostic Tests
- Laboratory panels Electrocardiogram (EKG), Chest x-ray (CXR)
- In elderly patients, do not forget an assessment of the preoperative status (pulmonary, cardiac, and renal evaluation if necessary preoperatively).

Upper gastrointestinal (UGI) series first maneuver—Lateral views are critical to visualize this posterior structure. Esophagogastroduodenoscopy (EGD) should not be done first, especially because EGD may perforate a Zenker's as two lumens will be visualized.

Open Diverticulectomy
- Make a left cervical incision over anterior border of sternocleidomastoid muscle (SCM).
- Diverticulum is located in the plane between the carotid sheath and trachea.
- Use a bougie in the esophagus to prevent narrowing when performing diverticulectomy with a TA stapler.

You may invert and perform a diverticulopexy to the precervical fascia in elderly and high-risk patients with diverticulums greater than 3 cm to reduce the risk of staple line leak, but the examiner will likely push you to perform resection.

You may leave it alone if it is less than 2 cm, although myotomy is still encouraged.

Always perform a cricopharyngeal myotomy—Gentle cephalad traction on the diverticulum will expose fibers

C. Sanders, D.O. (✉)
General Surgery, University of Medicine and Dentistry of New Jersey, School of Osteopathic Medicine, Stratford, NJ, USA
e-mail: cmsst93@msn.com

M.A. Neff (ed.), *Passing the General Surgery Oral Board Exam*,
DOI 10.1007/978-1-4614-7663-4_6, © Springer Science+Business Media New York 2014

of the cricopharngeus muscle, which are divided and bluntly dissected from the underlying mucosa and continued onto the esophagus for several centimeters. Always drain the incision.

Endoscopic Stapling

A candidate for endoscopic stapling must be able to undergo hyperextension of the neck.

Diverticula <2 cm or >5 cm are not good candidates for endoscopic repair.

A flexible endoscopy is performed.

Make sure you are in the true lumen.

The scope tends to pass preferentially into the diverticulum due to the tightness of the cricopharyngeous muscle.

A guide wire is then passed through the scope and into the stomach.

The flexible scope is removed and replaced with the rigid endoscope device.

The blade of the rigid scope passes into the true lumen and the diverticulum, exposing the septum between the two structures.

The diverticulum should be irrigated and sized.

A traction stitch is then placed in the septum using the endostitch.

An EndoGIA stapling device is then passed through the rigid endoscope to divide the septum.

The septum should be divided down to the bottom of the diverticula.

Multiple firings of the stapler may be required.

A completion flexible endoscopy should be performed to inspect the staple line and to make sure the entire septum has been divided.

Common Curveballs

Patient develops a postoperative leak or wound infection (open the incision to drain the wound infection or abscess that may develop following a leak)

Performing a diverticulopexy leads to perforation of the diverticulum (perforation of the cervical esophagus can generally be treated conservatively with restricted PO intake and antibiotics; the neck incision may be opened to drain any neck abscess that may develop)

Injury to the recurrent laryngeal nerve is identified postoperatively (Unilateral nerve injury may be asymptomatic or the patient may develop hoarseness. If the nerve has not been completely transected, symptoms will generally improve over time with therapy. Breathing problems are rare with unilateral injury. Transected nerves identified intraoperatively should be repaired. Injuries identified postoperatively are generally not immediately repaired. Repair of the damaged nerve is usually not attempted for at least 6 months if the patient's symptoms have not shown improvement.)

Diverticulectomy leads to narrowing of the esophagus after not using a bougie (balloon dilation or stenting may be attempted if the patient is symptomatic; if the stricture is identified outside of the early postoperative period, the stricture should be biopsied to rule out a cancer)

Injury to esophagus occurs intraoperatively (a primary repair should be performed; if a long segment of the cervical esophagus is involved, an SCM flap can be performed to reinforce the repair)

Clean Kills

Forgetting to leave a drain

Not describing the procedure properly

Forgetting to perform the cricopharyngeal myotomy

Forgetting to perform UGI or not performing prior to EGD

Discussing an endoscopic treatment that you have never seen (never describe an operation you have never performed; instead, say something like, "I do not perform this operation, but I know the key aspects are the following…")

Summary

Zenker's diverticulum is rare and occurs most commonly in the elderly (50 % in patients >70 years of age). It has been characterized as a disorder of diminished upper esophageal sphincter opening with increased hypopharyngeal pressure. The most common symptoms are dysphagia, regurgitation of undigested food particles, and halitosis. Recurrent upper respiratory infections from chronic aspirations can lead to life-threatening respiratory insufficiency.

A UGI series should be the first diagnostic test performed when a Zenker's diverticulum is suspected due to risk of perforation with EGD. One needs to be aware that more than 50 % of patients will present with complaints related to other upper gastrointestinal (GI) pathology. There is a particularly high association of this disorder with hiatal hernia and GERD. Thus, additional diagnostic studies such as EGD, manometry, and pH monitoring should be performed.

Traditionally, an open diverticulectomy has been the procedure of choice. However, in recent years, the endoscopic stapling technique has shown no increase in morbidity and is gaining favor as an alternative to an open procedure. Keep in mind that endoscopic stapling does not remove the diverticulum.

Achalasia

Concept

Achalasia features esophageal aperistalsis (loss of Auerbach's plexus), failure of the lower esophageal sphincter to relax, and resultant esophageal dilation.

Way Question May Be Asked?

"A 37-year-old woman presents on referral from her GI doctor with difficulty swallowing liquids and solids and substernal pain after meals for approximately 1 year."

Rarely will you be given the diagnosis on referral or shown the typical "bird's beak" UGI. Patients may also have aspiration or referral for a megaesophagus.

How to Answer?

You must be methodical in your approach to dysphagia because the scenario will end up being something you leave out. Differential diagnosis includes spasm, achalasia, stricture, and tumor (benign and malignant).

First, take a complete history, including risk factors for malignancy and the onset of the dysphagia.

Second, perform a complete physical examination including epigastric masses and lymph node basins. (These will all be negative but if you leave out the physical examination, the patient will end up having a pronounced supraclavicular node and the scenario will have changed to esophageal cancer with obvious metastases).

Appropriate preoperative studies include full laboratory panels, EKG, and CXR.

Appropriate workup of dysphagia always includes UGI, EGD (risk of malignancy increased in these patients), and manometry.

Treatment should also be stepwise with the following:

1. Attempts at medical therapy may include nitrates and calcium channel blockers.
2. Esophageal dilatation with pneumatic balloon under fluoroscopy to dilate and disrupt the fibers of the lower esophageal sphincter (LES; also be prepared for the scenario to switch to perforation here, which has ~4 % risk). Dilatation alone has approximately a 70 % response rate.

   Bougie dilation up to 54 Fr can also be performed, but symptom relief typically lasts only a few months.
3. BoTox injection with 80 units in four divided doses directed into the LES by endoscopy can be considered in older, debilitated patients.

4. Surgical myotomy can be done laparoscopically, thoracoscopically, or by an open transabdominal or transthoracic approach. Minimally invasive approaches are becoming the more popular methods of repair. However, this is not a commonly performed operation at most institutions. Describe the method of repair that you are most familiar with.

Procedure
   Left lateral approach (thoracic), supine (transabdominal)
   Double-lumen endotracheal tube (ETT; thoracic approach)
   Esophageal bougie
   Longitudinal myotomy from a point 1 cm onto gastric cardia to inferior pulmonary vein
   Muscle edges should separate by 1–2 cm
   ± Antireflux procedure (controversial but many surgeons will perform a partial wrap—Belsey, Dor, or Toupet)
   Postoperative UGI series with gastrograffin prior to feeding

Common Curveballs

Patient has a malignancy on endoscopy (perform a biopsy and proceed with metastatic workup; further management will be based off these results)

Patient does not have classic manometry (many unnamed motility disorders may affect the body of the esophagus and LES, so you may not see the classic findings of achalasia in the early part of the disease; if malignancy has been ruled out, medical therapy and dilation may be performed in an attempt at relief of symptoms)

Patient perforates after EGD (patient should be NPO with parenteral nutrition and antibiotics; primary repair should be performed with a muscle or pleural flap reinforcement as needed, and the distal esophageal perforations should be widely drained)

Patient has "megaesophagus" (need to rule out a distal malignancy causing proximal esophageal dilation vs. achalasia)

Patient has bad reflux if you didn't perform a wrap

Patient has bad pulmonary function tests (PFTs) and will not tolerate a thoracotomy (open or laparoscopic Heller myotomy may be performed by a transabdominal approach)

You perforate the esophagus performing the myotomy (repair with absorbable suture and cover with wrap)

Clean Kills

You forget the UGI, EGD, or manometry

You cannot describe the myotomy or forget to mention extending into stomach

You get stuck in referring patient back to the GI doc or in describing medical therapy and will not take the patient to the operating room (OR) for myotomy

Summary

Achalasia is a disorder in which the LES fails to relax. This leads to pressurization and dilation of the esophagus with progressive loss of peristalsis. Achalasia is also known to be a premalignant condition. Squamous cell cancer is the most common type, with an 8 % risk over a 20-year period.

The classic triad of symptoms for achalasia are dysphagia, regurgitation, and weight loss. Dysphagia is usually progressive from liquids to solids. Patients will usually describe havening to eat slowly and requiring large volumes of water to help wash down their food. Manometry is the criterion standard test for diagnosis. The pressure of the LES is greater than 35 mmHg and will fail to relax with swallowing. The pressure in the esophageal body will also be above baseline with no evidence of progressive peristalsis. UGI series shows a dilated esophagus, with the tapering in the distal esophagus referred to as the classic "bird's beak" appearance. There is also lack of a gastric air bubble on upright imaging. EGD must be performed to rule out a distal esophageal malignancy, which may mimic the typical findings seen on the UGI series.

Treatment strategies take a progressive approach and are aimed only at palliation of symptoms. Esophagomyotomy offers superior results and is less traumatic than balloon dilation. A modified Heller myotomy is the operation of choice and can be performed by open or laparoscopic technique.

Esophageal Cancer

Concept

Esophageal cancer is one of the leading causes of cancer deaths. Squamous cell has traditionally accounted for the majority of esophageal cancers, although the frequency of adenocarcinoma is increasing. Risk factors include achalasia, Barrett's esophagus, caustic injuries, diverticula, leukoplakia, Plummer-Vinson syndrome, smoking, and alcohol use.

Way Question May Be Asked?

"A 61-year-old male smoker presents to your office with a new onset of dysphagia. On review of systems, the patient has lost 15 pounds in the last month and the dysphagia is worse for solids compared to liquids."

Be careful of the adult patient that presents with an esophageal stricture—you must rule out malignancy with both biopsy and brushing of the stricture for cytology.

How to Answer?

Complete history and physical examination (weight loss, vomiting, palpable mass, risk factors, check for supraclavicular node, enlarged liver)
Laboratory tests (full laboratory panels, preoperative nutritional status)
Appropriate diagnostic tests:
   UGI series
   Endoscopy and biopsy
   Bronchoscopy (if cancer is in upper two-thirds of esophagus to rule out esophagobronchial fistula)
   Computed tomography (CT) scan of the chest and abdomen (enlarged lymph nodes, celiac/mediastinal, metastases to liver/lungs)
   Endoscopic ultrasound may be used to provide more accurate staging of tumor invasion and regional node status
   Barium enema/colonoscopy may be performed if the colon is a possible conduit (you do not need a preoperative angiogram)
Be complete, but do not dwell on these because the examiner is trying to get to more complicated issues, such as the indications for surgery/palliation, performance of the surgery, and management of complications after surgery. You can discuss preoperative nutrition with jejunostomy tube (J-tube) feeds or total parenteral nutrition (TPN), but it must be at least 2 weeks in duration preoperatively to see any benefit.
   Contraindications for resection:
Metastatic disease (must perform fine needle aspiration [FNA] to prove it is metastatic)
Enlarged mediastinal/paratracheal/celiac nodes
Fistula to the airway
   Nonsurgical palliation:
Metallic stents
Laser fulguration
Feeding tubes
Intraluminal tubes
Chemotherapy/radiotherapy

Surgical Treatment

Be able to describe a Ivor-Lewis procedure or transhiatal procedure.
Remember that cervical anastomosis is safer than intrathoracic.

Any transhiatal procedure might need to be converted to thoracotomy if the tumor is fixed to adjacent structures.

You can perform anastomosis as running or interrupted, single or double layer (staplers are associated with increased risk of stenosis)

If you are performing a thoracotomy, remember preoperative tests (PFTs)

The stomach is the best organ to replace the esophagus with.

Send to pathology to check intraoperative margins.

Perform postoperative UGI series on day 5–7 depending on preference.

Maintain chest tube/J-tube.

Key Features of the Ivor-Lewis Procedure:

Perform abdominal portion first, then right posterolateral thoracotomy

Abdominal exploration

Create gastric tube

Preserve right gastric and right gastroepiploic

Kocher maneuver to allow gastric pull-up

Pyloroplasty/pyloromyotomy

Double lumen tube to deflate right lung

Intrathoracic anastomosis

Left thoracoabdominal incision may be made for distal esophageal carcinomas

Key Features of Transhiatal Procedure:

Abdominal and left neck incision

Be prepared to do thoracotomy

Blunt mediastinal dissection

Order: abdominal/cervical/mediastinal/anastomosis

Common Curveballs

Cancer presents as a new stricture in an adult

Patient has anastomotic leak (patient may become septic or it may be a silent leak only seen on postoperative UGI series; management will depend on whether it is in the chest or the neck)

There is necrosis of the gastric tube (the mediastinum should be drained; you may need to perform a partial or total resection of the gastric tube with a diversion procedure and feeding tube)

Saliva comes out of the chest tube (leak as described above)

Examiner asks you to describe diversion for total disruption of anastomosis postoperatively (the cervical esophagus is brought out through the neck or chest as an ostomy; requires placement of a feeding J-tube)

Patient has postoperative fever (monitor for leak/sepsis)

Examiner asks you how to boost nutritional status preoperatively (placement of a feeding gastrostomy or jejunostomy tube [preferred] or parenteral nutrition; nutritional support must be started weeks before the planned procedure)

Patient develops a chylothorax (50 % resolve spontaneously. Use a chest tube to drain the pleural space. Start parenteral nutrition or fat-restricted diet with medium chain fatty acids; administer Octreotide. Lymphangiography or Evans blue dye can be used to localize the leak. Persistent leak may require thoracic duct ligation between 8th and 12th rib on right via thoracotomy or thoracoscopy.)

Patient has delayed gastric emptying postoperatively (can occur despite pyloromyotomy and pyloroplasty; administer erythromycin, injection of Botox, and balloon dilation or stent placement across the pyloris)

Patient has recurrent laryngeal nerve injury during the surgery

Examiner asks about management of a late anastomotic stricture (balloon or bougie dilation is usually effective)

Examiner asks about neoadjuvant chemotherapy/radiotherapy (depends on the type of cancer, location and extent of disease)

Patient has features suggestive of unresectability (evidence of liver or lung metastases; invasion into the membranous trachea, left main stem bronchus, or aorta; metastases to the mesentery or aortic nodes; peritoneal or omental metastases)

Patient has injury to trachea during cervical or thoracic dissection (it is usually to the membranous portion of the trachea and you can usually advance ETT, So that the balloon of the ETT is positioned distal to the tear and then perform repair; may need to split upper sternum to accomplish)

Suture Line Recurrence

Radiation ± chemotherapy

Repeat resection

Check frozen section of esophageal margin before making anastomosis

If a positive celiac node found during surgery, then what (this is unresectable disease)?

This should be assessed prior to any resection performed. If a positive celiac or mesenteric node is found, the plan for resection should be aborted with treatment goal aimed at palliation rather than cure. Palliative measures include radiation ± chemotherapy, dilation, laser and photodynamic therapy, stent placement, and feeding gastrostomy or jejunostomy tube.

Clean Kills

Not treating a stricture as a possible malignancy and performing simply an antireflux procedure

Placing gastrostomy tube for preoperative nutrition and destroying potential gastric tube

Trying to resect someone with obvious evidence of nonresectability

Not performing pyloroplasty/pyloromyotomy with gastric pull-up

Not being able to describe the operation

Not knowing nonoperative methods of palliation

Not being able to manage the possible complications of your procedure

Summary

Esophageal cancer is the sixth most common malignancy in the United States. Squamous cell cancer is the most common type worldwide; however, 70 % of patients in the United States have adenocarcinoma. Risk factors include age >65 years, male sex, smoking, heavy alcohol use, GERD, obesity, and Barrett's esophagus. Symptoms will vary depending on the stage of presentation. Early-stage cancers are asymptomatic or patients typically present with symptoms of GERD, such as heartburn and indigestion. Dysphagia and weight loss are most commonly associated with late-stage cancers. Symptoms of systemic metastasis include jaundice, pain from bone metastasis, and shortness of breath.

Diagnostic workup includes UGI series and EGD with biopsy. Endoscopic ultrasound can be used to further evaluate the depth and length of invasion, as well as involvement of adjacent structures and lymph nodes, along with performance of FNA. The use of positron emission tomography (PET) scan to evaluate for metastatic disease is debatable. The sensitivity and specificity of PET scan exceeds that of CT scan for distant metastatic disease and its use upstages approximately 20 % of cancers. However, it cannot be used to determine the depth of invasion and it is difficult to differentiate regional lymph node disease from the primary tumor. Thoracoscopy and laparoscopy are highly accurate for staging, although they are rather invasive methods of assessing nodal status.

Treatment strategies will vary depending upon the type of cancer, location, and stage of disease. Methods of treatment include surgery, chemotherapy, radiation, or a combination of these modalities. No combination has been proven superior. Squamous cell cancer is far more sensitive to chemotherapy than is esophageal adenocarcinoma.

Esophagectomy either via an open or minimally invasive thoracic or transhiatal approach should be performed in all patients without evidence of metastatic disease. A gastric pull up is the preferred conduit for reconstruction if not extensively involved with the tumor and a 5-cm margin can be obtained. Care must be taken to preserve the right gastric and gastroepiploic arteries to preserve blood supply to the conduit. Alternatively, a colonic (typically left colon) or jejunal interposition can be used. These conduits are associated with a higher morbidity because three separate anastomoses are required to use a colon conduit and the jejunal vascular supply limits its mobility and length.

Esophageal Perforation

Concept

Esophageal perforation is a potentially lethal condition that may be spontaneous (Boerhaave's syndrome) or result from trauma, swallowed foreign bodies, ingestion of caustic substances, malignancy, or iatrogenic (nasogastric tube [NGT]/endoscopy). The most common cause today is iatrogenic related to endoscopic maneuvers (biopsy/dilatations/cautery).

Way Question May Be Asked?

"A 28-year-old man presents to the emergency department with acute onset of epigastric/chest pain after several episodes of vomiting from alcohol abuse."

The patient may also present after dilatation of stricture, achalasia, biopsy for Barrett's esophagus, dysplasia, or malignancy. Rarely will the examiner mention any of the following: crepitance in the suprasternal notch, diminished breath sounds in the left chest, a left pleural effusion or air in the mediastinum on CXR, or triad of vomiting/low thoracic pain/cervical emphysema.

How to Answer?

As usual, perform a complete history and physical examination, but also make an assessment of the stability of the patient. A patient in shock needs urgent treatment.

History
  Previous esophageal disorders
  Any history of ulcer disease
  Pancreatitis
  Heart disease
  Ingestions
  Timing of pain to vomiting

Physical Examination
  Vital signs
  Cervical examination (subcutaneous emphysema occurs more with cervical perforations), diminished breath sounds in left chest

Diagnostic Tests

Full laboratory panels (amylase to rule out pancreatitis)

EKG (to rule out myocardial infarction)

CXR (pleural effusion, hydropneumothorax, mediastinal air)

Lateral neck x-ray (subcutaneous emphysema)

A gastrograffin swallow should identify leak. If not, you may then get a barium swallow. (Gastrograffin is used before barium to avoid mediastinitis.)

Do not perform an endoscopy!

Treatment should also be stepwise with consideration given to the following:

Time since perforation

Location/size of the perforation

Patient's overall clinical status

Degree of contamination

Underlying esophageal disorder (Barrett's esophagus/malignancy)

All patients should receive nothing by mouth (NPO), broad-spectrum antibiotics, and NGT.

Nonoperative therapy is only for patients with walled-off small perforations, minimal symptoms, and no sepsis, with frequent reassessments and a low threshold for surgery.

Once taken to OR, all patients get same basic plan:

Debridement

Closure (of perforation)

Drainage

1. If it is within 24 h of perforation, attempt primary repair.

    (a) For perforations in the upper two-thirds of the esophagus, perform a right thoracotomy (sixth or seventh intercostal space), debridement of all nonviable tissue, myotomy to define extent of mucosal injury, closure in two layers over the NGT, cover with tissue flap (pleural/pericardium/intercostal muscle), and place a chest tube. Patient is then kept NPO, on TPN or enteral feeds through gastrostomy or J-tube, and continued on antibiotics.

    (b) For a perforation in the lower third of the esophagus, perform a left thoracotomy (seventh or eighth intercostal space) by the same procedure as above, with the ability to now cover repair with Thal patch, diaphragm muscle, and fundoplication.

    (c) For a perforation in the abdominal esophagus, perform an upper midline with a low threshold to making a left thoracotomy (make sure to prepare the left chest) and cover repair with fundoplication.

    (d) For a cervical perforation, make an incision in the left neck along the SCM (unless the perforation is clearly visualized in the right neck).

    The SCM and carotid sheath are retracted laterally. The middle thyroidal vein and omohyoid muscle are divided and the trachea and esophagus are retracted medially.

You need to bluntly dissect the tissue posterior to the esophagus to assess whether there are infection tracts in the mediastinum.

Cervical perforations can be difficult to locate for primary repair.

The neck may be loosely closed and drained with a JP drain or the incision may be left open and packed depending upon the extent of contamination.

2. If the patient is unstable after 24 h, perform an esophageal exclusion:

    (a) Debridement of mediastinum/esophagus/lung

    (b) Establish effective drainage with two chest tubes

    (c) Leave esophagus open

    (d) Ligate gastroesophageal junction (GEJ) with two ties of no. 2 chromic

    (e) Place NGT above the perforation

    (f) Perform high-volume irrigation through the NGT

    (g) Patient should be NPO/TPN or have J-tube feeds/antibiotics

        or

    (c) Segmental esophagectomy

    (d) Gastrostomy/J-tube

    (e) Cervical esophagostomy

    (f) NPO/TPN or J-tube feeds/antibiotics

3. Esophageal resection is appropriate if there exists pathology in the esophageal wall. This is delayed if the patient is unstable. It can be performed immediately with the stomach and a left cervical anastomosis.

    Perform a postoperative UGI series with gastrograffin prior to feeding once there is resolution of sepsis and repair has chance to heal.

Common Curveballs

No leak is seen on gastrograffin swallow (repeat test with barium)

CXR/neck x-ray are negative

Patient is unstable (proceed to operative exploration)

Location of the leak changes after you suggest an algorithm

Time to detection of the leak changes after you suggest an algorithm

Examiner pushes you towards nonoperative therapy

Nonoperative therapy fails

Patient has a leak after your repair (esophageal diversion)

Patient has a perforation during dilatation of achalasia or during examination of Barrett's esophagus (esophagectomy is appropriate here, and you may proceed with gastric reconstruction if there is limited contamination; for patients without end-stage achalasia, a primary repair with a contralateral myotomy followed by fundoplication may be performed)

Clean Kills

Performing endoscopy to identify leak (and spread infection/ create tension pneumothorax)

Not using water-soluble contrast enema

Attempting to perform immediate resection/reconstruction with unprepped colon

Not ruling out distal obstruction

Not attempting primary repair on early perforation

Not ruling out myocardial infarction, pancreatitis, perforated peptic ulcer disease (PUD), and aortic dissection.

Summary

The goals when dealing with a potential esophageal perforation are early recognition, hemodynamic support, antibiotics, drainage, repair, and nutritional support. Operative management is required in most cases to reduce patient morbidity and mortality. Nonoperative management is acceptable only for patients with minimal contamination.

The optimal treatment for esophageal perforation is primary repair. However, primary repair should not be performed when the patient is unstable, the perforation is too large, or in the setting of an esophageal malignancy, end-stage benign disease, and severe diffuse mediastinitis. In these circumstances, the patient will likely require an esophageal resection. Furthermore, perforations in the cervical esophagus may be difficult to assess to perform a primary repair. Although use of esophageal stents have been described for treating esophageal perforations, this is not standard of care and there are no established guidelines on patient selection.

Distal obstruction should be ruled out before any repair is performed. Devitalized tissue should be debrided. A longitudinal myotomy should be done to assess the extent of mucosal injury. Repair occurs in two layers. A muscle, pleural, or omental flap can be used to reinforce the repair. A fundal wrap can also serve as a method of reinforcement for lower esophageal perforations.

Nutrition support is important. Feeding tubes may not be necessary in well-nourished patients with small perforations and limited contamination. For those patients with poor nutritional status, diffuse contamination, and sepsis, a feeding jejunostomy tube is preferred. Most patients are kept NPO for a minimum of 7 days prior to obtaining an UGI series. If there is no evidence of leak, the NGT can be removed and the patient is started on enteral feeding. J-tube feeds can be initiated within the first few postoperative days. Chest tubes are typically removed only after the patient has been tolerating enteral feeding without continued evidence of leak.

Esophageal Varices

Concept

Esophageal varices are a life-threatening complication of portal hypertension. The major questions are often about stabilizing these patients and knowing the appropriate timing for surgical intervention. Also, make sure to rule out other potential sources for upper gastrointestinal bleeding (UGIB).

Way Question May Be Asked?

"A 51-year-old man presents to the emergency department with three episodes of massive hemoptysis. His social history is remarkable for extensive alcohol abuse and his past medical history is remarkable for multiple admissions for alcoholic pancreatitis."

The patient may be referred to you with the diagnosis of bleeding varices from another hospital, or it may be simply a patient with an UGIB.

How to Answer?

Perform a brief, focused history and physical examination while resuscitating the patient.

History
  Alcohol use
  Episodes of encephalopathy, bleeding varices
  History of pancreatitis
  History of PUD
  (Be sure to do all this while resuscitating the patient or you will have great history on a dead patient!)

Physical Examination
  Stigmata of liver disease
  Ascites

Resuscitation
  Intravenous (IV) access, central venous pressure line, laboratory panels (especially coagulation), Type and cross (T+C), transfusion of packed red blood cells and fresh frozen plasma
  NGT, lavage stomach

Treatment

You can consider a Sengstaken-Blakemore tube after intubating the patient (be prepared to describe technique!)

Start vasopressin drip 0.4 U/min (add IV nitroglycerin if patient has a history of coronary artery disease and consider Swan Ganz Catheter (SGC))

Start IV somatostatin (25 μg/h)

Use a beta blocker to lower heart rate (HR) if it is not lower than 100; target HR is 55–60 or a decrease in resting HR by 25 % (administer slowly as it may precipitously drop systolic blood pressure; titration to goal HR may take days)

(In the back of your mind, you should be considering Child's class because Child's C patients need a liver transplantation; i.e., bilirubin >3, albumin <3, severe ascites)

Endoscopy (once hemodynamically stabilized)

At EGD, you can consider sclerotherapy and banding. (However, neither will be available or will work!)

If EGD fails, you can consider transjugular intrahepatic portosystemic shunt (TIPS):

Functions as a side to side portal caval shunt

Good for refractory variceal bleeds and ascites

The hepatic vein is accessed through an internal jugular approach and tunnel then created to the portal vein. A coated stent is then placed across the tract to decease portal pressure below 12 mmHg (However, TIPS wont be available and will need consider indications for surgical shunt procedure).

Surgery Indications: Uncontrolled Bleeding

Emergency portosystemic shunt

Mesocaval—8-mm PTFE shunt between the superior mesenteric vein (SMV) and inferior vena cava (IVC)

Identify the middle colic vein and follow distally to the SMV (to the right of the superior mesenteric artery). Identify the IVC through the right colonic mesentery adjacent to the duodenum. Anastomose to the IVC first, then to the side of the SMV (can use left internal jugular vein if there is a contaminated field). This shunt does not dissect in the porta hepatis so it does not compromise the potential for a future liver transplantation.

Other Choices

Gastric devascularization

End-to-end anastomosis limited esophagectomy with ligation of the left gastric vein

Gastrostomy and suture ligation

Common Curveballs

Patient has UGIB secondary to PUD, esophagitis, and gastric varices

Bleeding continues postoperatively

Patient becomes encephalopathic postoperatively check electroencephalogram [high amplitude, low frequency, triphasic waves, but not specific]; check CT/MRI to rule out intracranial lesion; start lactulose and rifaximin; re-evaluate shunt)

Patient had prior abdominal surgery

Patient is Child's class C (liver transplantation is best option)

Patient aspirates or perforates after balloon tamponade

In case of aspiration, start antibiotics to cover pneumonia.

Perforation can occur from missed placement of Blakemore tube or necrosis from balloon tamponade.

You can attempt conservative management with a chest tube because patient will likely be too unstable for an operative procedure [high mortality].)

May need esophagectomy

Patient has thrombosed splenic vein and bleeding gastric varices (needs only a splenectomy)

Patient develops hepatic failure or hepatorenal syndrome postoperatively

The same pharmacologic support with the addition of dopamine is initiated for supportive measures.

Patient should be evaluated for liver transplantation.

Dialysis may be necessary and can be used as supportive measure until transplant available. There is no role for shunts as a treatment measure.)

Examiner asks you to describe other shunting procedures

Clean Kills

Performing a distal splenorenal shunt

Not being able to describe your surgical procedure

Describing the Sugiura procedure (you do not want to describe something you have never done before, and this procedure is rarely done in the United States)

Rushing to the operating room

Not performing an EGD/trying sclerotherapy/banding

Not knowing how to use a Sengstaken–Blakemore tube

Not resuscitating the patient properly

Summary

The mortality rate for an acute variceal bleed can be as high as 50 % and is based on failure to control hemorrhage and re-bleeding. The biggest risk factor for mortality and early re-bleeding is the severity of liver disease. The most important measures to reduce early mortality are effective resuscitation with correction of hypovolemia, prompt identification, and control.

EGD is the most common method of detecting varices. Ultrasound is used to look for splenomegaly and portal venous thrombosis as evidence for portal hypertension

(HTN). It is also important to realize that 25–50 % of patients with portal HTN will have upper gastrointestinal bleeding from something other than varices. EGD should be performed once the patient has been resuscitated. Intubation may be necessary for airway protection due to encephalopathy and risk of aspiration from massive hematemesis. A Sengstaken–Blakemore tube can be used as a method to slow or stop variceal bleeding to assist with resuscitation efforts and temporize bleeding enough so that the source can be identified on EGD. It can also aid in diagnosis if placed properly, because blood will continue to be visualized from the gastric aspirate in the presence of bleeding from gastric varices.

Endoscopic methods for treating esophageal varices include variceal banding and sclerotherapy. In addition, efforts need to be made to lower portal venous pressure. Pharmacologic agents used to decrease splanchnic blood flow in the acute setting include vasopressin analogues, somatostatin, and nonselective beta-blockers (nadolol, propranolol). Nitrates are also effective to lower portal pressures, but they are not well tolerated by patients. All patients should also be placed on antibiotics because 20 % of patients with variceal bleeding and cirrhosis will develop spontaneous bacterial peritonitis.

The surgical approach to the treatment of portal HTN includes portosystemic shunts, esophageal transection, gastroesophageal devascularization, and liver transplantation. Surgical procedures are rarely performed now due to the efficacy of liver transplantation. Patients with Child's class A cirrhosis and portal HTN secondary to portal venous thrombosis are the best candidates for non-transplant operations.

Gastroesophageal Reflux Disease

Concept

GERD is caused by incompetent lower esophageal sphincter related to inadequate pressure (<6 mmHg), inadequate length (<2 cm), and insufficient intraabdominal esophagus (<1 cm). Hiatal hernia, delayed gastric emptying, and bile reflux may complicate the picture.

Way Question May Be Asked?

"A 45-year-old man presents to your office with a history of heartburn, choking at night, and recent onset of asthma."

Symptoms may be many and include chest pain, water brash, adult-onset asthma, dysphagia, odynophagia, sinusitis, aspiration pneumonia, choking feeling at night, regurgitation, excessive salivation, and chronic hoarseness. Also, the patient may present with a complication of their reflux disease: Barrett's esophagus, stricture, or ulcer.

How to Answer?

You must be methodical in your approach to not get caught by the patient with abnormal motility who you decide to perform a complete wrap on.

First, take a complete history, including relationship to meals, to solids versus liquids, to any maneuvers tried (loose clothing, caffeine cessation, trial of H2 blockers or proton pump inhibitors).

Second, perform a complete physical examination, including epigastric masses and lymph node basins. (All will be negative, but if you leave out the physical examination, the patient will end up having a pronounced supraclavicular node and the scenario will have switched to esophageal cancer with obvious metastases.)

Obtain the appropriate preoperative studies, including full laboratory panels, EKG, and CXR.

Perform the appropriate workup of GERD, which always starts with a barium UGI series.

Look for reflux, hernia, shortened esophagus, diverticula, and other motility disorders.

The next test should be an upper endoscopy to evaluate the severity of the reflux:

Stage I: Erythema and edema

Stage II: Ulcerations

Stage III: Stricture

The rest of the workup must include the following:

Manometry to rule out ineffective motility that will affect your type of antireflux procedure, to document the low LES pressures, and determine the location of the LES

24-h pH monitoring to document the relationship between patient's symptoms and reflux as well as provide a baseline for postoperative evaluation of success of surgery

(A gastric emptying study should be added for any patient with a history of significant belching or bloating after meals and/or history of duodenal ulcer because a delay in gastric emptying contributes to 10 % of Nissen failures.)

Remember the indications for surgery are
failure of medical therapy or
complications of reflux disease.
(Young age is a relative indication.)

Procedure
Assuming normal motility, perform a Nissen fundoplication (today usually performed laparoscopically) as follows:
Lithotomy position
5–6 ports

Nissen performed over a bougie (54–56)

Start dissection at gastrohepatic ligament

Mobilize esophagus well into mediastinum

Divide short gastrics down one-third along greater curve

Crural repair

3-cm anterior wrap

Take care not to injure the vagus nerve, perforate the stomach or esophagus, injure the spleen, or make the wrap too tight, too long, or twist the stomach when passing it around esophagus.

Belsey, Dor, or Toupet can be performed in patients with ineffective esophageal motility.

Obtain a postoperative UGI series with gastrograffin prior to feeding.

Common Curveballs

Patient has a malignancy, Barrett's esophagus, or stricture on endoscopy (nondilatable stricture = surgery)

Patient does not have classic manometry

Perforation occurs during the procedure by advancing bougie or postoperatively on UGI series (perform primary repair and cover with wrap if distal; may attempt conservative management if small and minimal contamination)

Patient presents with a stricture where first you must rule out malignancy and dilate prior to any studies

Patient has "shortened esophagus" (be prepared to describe Collis gastroplasty)

Patient develops pneumothorax or bleeding from liver/spleen during procedure

Perforation of esophagus occurs during the procedure or pre-operative workup (scenario switch)

Fundoplication herniates into chest postoperatively (poor hiatal closure, did not mobilize esophagus enough)

Fundoplication falls apart postoperatively (technical failure)

Patient has "gas bloat" syndrome postoperatively (inadequate gastric emptying that may improve with time; consider pyloroplasty or conversion to partial wrap)

Patient has difficulty swallowing postoperatively (made wrap too tight)

Clean Kills

You forget the UGI, EGD, or manometry

You cannot describe the fundoplication or forget to mention taking the short gastrics

You take the patient to surgery right away without trying medical therapy

You do not take an adequate history and perform a Nissen on a patient with achalasia

Discussing endoscopic measures to treat Barrett's esophagus (cryotherapy or phototherapy)

Discussing endoscopic measures to treat GERD (Plicator, Stretta, or newly approved injectable agents)

Summary

GERD affects 20–40 % of the population. GERD is largely due to incompetence of the LES. Additional contributing factors include presence of a hiatal hernia, delayed gastric emptying, and decreased esophageal motility. Symptoms include heartburn, substernal chest pain, dysphagia, cough, increased salivation, and asthma-like symptoms.

Diagnosis is based off of clinical suspicion and confirmed with 24-h pH monitoring. Additional test include barium swallow, EGD, and manometry. Biopsies should be taken in patients with long-standing or refractory disease to rule out Barrett's esophagus or adenocarcinoma.

Treatment consists of lifestyle modifications such as weight loss, smaller meals, smoking cessation, eating several hours before bedtime, and elevating the head of the bed. H2 blockers are effective in approximately 50 % of patients. The most successful medications are proton pump inhibitors. Nissen fundoplication is reserved for patients who are noncompliant with or fail medical therapy. Five to eight centimeters of intra-abdominal esophagus is necessary to perform a successful 3–5 cm fundoplication to prevent reflux. The fundoplication can be performed over a bougie to help prevent the wrap from being too tight. If the esophagus is short and intra-abdominal esophageal length is inadequate, a lengthening procedure such as the collis gastroplasty should be performed. A partial fundoplication (e.g., Dor, Toupet) should be considered for patients with motility disorders to avoid significant dysphagia.

Hiatal Hernia

Concept

There are four types of hiatal hernias:

I. Sliding hernia, GEJ in chest

II. Paraesophageal, GEJ in abdomen

III. Type II with shortening of esophagus and GEJ in chest

IV. Additional abdominal organs (spleen, colon) in hernia defect

Board questions seem to focus on the treatment of type II and III paraesophageal hernias that are symptomatic.

Way Question May Be Asked?

"A 53 y/o male presents to the hospital with abdominal pain. On futher evaluation, his chief complaint is right sided abdominal and flank pain and he has noticed a red color to his urine. What's your management?"

The patient may also have postprandial pain, which may not be related to any specific solid or liquid foods. Pain is likely epigastric.

How to Answer?

Take a complete history and perform a physical examination (you may have been given all this information already).

History
    Character of pain
    Relation to meals
    Relation to solids/liquids
    Previous esophageal problems/diagnoses
    Heartburn
    Dysphagia
    Vomiting
    Anemia
    Early satiety
Physical Examination
    Abdominal masses
    Lymphadenopathy
Diagnostic Tests
    Usual laboratory panels (check hemoglobin and hematocrit because often patients are anemic)
    CXR (may see gastric bubble behind heart shadow)
    Barium swallow
    Upper endoscopy (examine for ulcerations, malignancies, diverticula)
    Manometry (helpful before deciding what degree of wrap to perform)

Indications for Surgery All paraesophageal hernias get surgery.
    Volvulus
    Ulcerations
    Anemia

Surgical Procedure
    Abdominal incision (can consider thoracic if you believe the patient has a shortened esophagus or prior abdominal operations)
    Reduction of stomach (herniated contents) and inspection
    Excision of hernia sac
    Closure of diaphragmatic defect (interrupted, nonabsorbable sutures)
    Anchoring stomach (Stamm gastrostomy or gastropexy to abdominal wall or to arcuate ligament)
    "Floppy" Nissen (unless severely abnormal manometry)

Common Curveballs

Patient has a malignancy on endoscopy
Patient has a shortened esophagus (Collis gastroplasty)
Patient has a mass on UGI series
Incarcerated contents (stomach) are strangulated and need resection
You cannot close crura without the use of a mesh
Patient has abnormal manometry so you cannot perform a 360-degree Nissen wrap
Examiner asks if it is necessary to perform an antireflux procedure
Patient has a pneumothorax from dissection of adhesions from sac to pleura
Patient has postoperative recurrence of hernia
Examiner asks how tight to reapproximate the crura
Patient has injury to stomach or esophagus during procedure (scenario switch)

Clean Kills

You forget the UGI or EGD
You forget to anchor the stomach or perform a wrap
You try to treat the patient medically/nonoperatively once you have diagnosed a paraesophageal hernia
You treat your patient with strangulation in the hernia sac as having angina or a myocardial infarction

Summary

Hiatal hernia involves the protrusion of intra-abdominal contents through an enlarged esophageal hiatus of the diaphragm. The incidence of hiatal hernia increases with age, with greater than 60 % of the population having a hiatal hernia after the age of 50 years. Risk factors

include obesity, increased intra-abdominal pressure from various conditions, and a previous hiatal operation. Symptoms commonly include heartburn, dysphagia, hoarseness, asthma, chest pain, or hematemesis, or a combination of these.

The diagnosis of hiatal hernia is made by UGI or EGD. A CXR may provide a clue to the diagnosis by the presence of a gas bubble behind the cardiac silhouette. Manometry should also be completed to rule out a motility disorder, which will help determine what type of wrap should be performed if pursuing surgical repair.

Treatment depends on the patient's symptoms and the anatomic configuration of the hernia. The majority of hiatal hernias are of the sliding type. Uncomplicated sliding hiatal hernias are treated symptomatically with medical therapy, although some patients may select surgical therapy. Complicated hiatal hernias (those with bleeding, volvulus, or obstruction) have a stronger indication for surgical repair.

Key components of the repair include complete reduction of the hernia sac, adequate mobilization of the esophagus, a tension-free crural repair, and loose Fundoplication. A partial fundoplication is considered with the additional presence of a motility disorder. A relaxing incision may need to be performed to allow for tension-free approximation of the crura.

Considerations for mesh placement include large hernia defects, recurrent hernias, and morbidly obese patients. Gastropexy should also be considered for those patients when there is a large hernia defect and the majority of the stomach is found in the intrathoracic position.

Genitourinary

Marc A. Neff

Renal Mass

Concept

This is an unusual question, but it is more important in everyday surgical life. There are a variety of renal masses, including abscesses, cysts, benign tumors, and malignancies (primary and metastatic). Look for suggestive history. Do not fall prey to percutaneous biopsy of suspected malignancy, and do not confuse with an adrenal lesion!

How to Answer?

History
  Flank pain
  Hematuria
  Fever, chills
  Family history of renal cell carcinoma (RCC)
  Prior malignancy (lung or breast cancer can metastasize to the kidney)
  New varicocele
  Hypercalcemia
  Tuberous sclerosis
  Renal insufficiency
Physical Examination
  Unlikely to feel the mass
  Varicocele
  Evidence of metastatic disease
Diagnostic Tests
  Complete labs, chest x-ray (CXR), urinalysis

Intravenous pyelogram—usually the first test to evaluate a patient with hematuria
Ultrasound—can determine if cystic or solid, can evaluate for a simple cysts with no septa or calcifications (these can be symptomatic but almost always benign)
Computed tomography (CT)—can evaluate solid lesion, inspect renal vein and inferior vena cava (IVC), look for metastatic lesions
Magnetic resonance imaging—if there is any doubt about IVC thrombus
CT-guided needle biopsy—rarely done for solid lesions due to risk of bleeding and tumor seeding
Angiogram—preoperative embolization of large lesions is a consideration

Surgery

Dependent on lesion
RCC gets radical nephrectomy
Transitional cell carcinoma (TCC) gets radical nephroureterectomy
However, do not go into describing these—say you would refer the patient to a urologist
Make sure to assess renal function and contribution from the side you are planning to remove—patient may need postoperative hemodialysis

Common Curveballs

Lesion is cystic with internal echoes/septae
Patient needs postoperative hemodialysis
Lesion will be TCC if you do not rule it out with ureteroscopy/biopsy
Patient bleeds from any percutaneous biopsy attempt
Patient is symptomatic from a simple cystic lesion (just need to unroof)
Patient actually has an adrenal lesion (scenario switch!)

M.A. Neff, M.D., F.A.C.S. (✉)
Minimally Invasive, 2201 Chapel Avenue West, Suite 100, Cherry Hill, NJ 08002, USA
e-mail: mneffyhs@aol.com

M.A. Neff (ed.), *Passing the General Surgery Oral Board Exam*,
DOI 10.1007/978-1-4614-7663-4_7, © Springer Science+Business Media New York 2014

Clean Kills

Offering laparoscopic kidney resection

Performing percutaneous biopsy of a solid lesion

Not referring the patient to a urologist (at least try before taking on such a case outside of your specialty)

Not ruling out metastatic disease

Not checking for possible lung/breast cancer with metastases to kidney

Performing radical nephrectomy only for TCC

Scrotal Mass

Concept

On the board examination, this is most likely to be a testicular mass. However, do not forget that hydrocele, varicocele, inguinal hernia, testicular torsion, and spermatoceles can all present as scrotal masses. Important points for your differential diagnosis are whether the mass is painful and whether it transilluminates.

Way Question May Be Asked?

"You are called to the emergency department to evaluate a 27-year-old male resident who has noticed a 2-cm mass in his left testicle. What do you do?" The age group most at risk is young males.

How to Answer?

History
    Pain (timing)
    Hernia
    Does patient perform his own testicular examinations?
Physical Examination
    Hernia
    Transillumination
    Tenderness
    Lymphadenopathy
Diagnostic Tests
    Alphafetoprotein (AFP), human chorionic gonadotropin (HCG), lactate dehydrogenase (LDH)

CXR (to rule out metastatic disease)
Ultrasound of the scrotum (all patients)
CT scan (to look for para-aortic lymph node enlargement)

Surgical Treatment

1. Inguinal orchiectomy (control spermatic cord early to minimize tumor spread)
2. Seminoma (HCG-human chorionic gonadotropin)
   (a) If markers are negative and there is minimal enlargement of the para-aortic nodes, then the patient should receive
       radiation to the para-aortic and ipsilateral pelvic nodes.
   (b) If there are bulky retroperitoneal nodes, positive markers, or distant metastases, then the patient should receive
       platinum-based chemotherapy.
3. Nonseminomatous tumors (embryonal, teratoma, teratocarcinoma, choriocarcinoma)
   (a) Perform retroperitoneal lymph node dissection followed by chemotherapy unless there are enlarged retroperitoneal nodes, then the patient should receive chemotherapy first.
   (b) Chemotherapy regimen is bleomycin, etopside, and platinum.

Common Curveballs

Scenario changes from seminoma or nonseminomatous tumor

Patient has enlarged retroperitoneal nodes on CT

Patient has evidence of metastatic disease

Patient has postoperative ejaculatory dysfunction

Tumor markers are positive

Clean Kills

Not performing <u>inguinal</u> orchiectomy

Not ordering tumor markers

Not knowing that seminoma is very radiosensitive

Not knowing what to do for para-aortic lymph nodes

Not performing a CT scan to evaluate the retroperitoneum

Hepatobiliary

Linda Szczurek and Marc A. Neff

Gallstone Ileus

Concept

Gallstone ileus is a mechanical obstruction in the terminal ileum from a large gallstone that has eroded through the gallbladder into the duodenum (cholecystoenteric fistula). It is seen in elderly patients with small bowel obstruction (SBO) who have no hernia and no previous surgeries. The stone is most commonly stuck at the terminal ileum/ileocecal valve.

Way Question May Be Asked?

"A 74-year-old woman is seen in the emergency department (ED) for a small bowel obstruction. Obstruction series confirms the small bowel obstruction with air in the biliary tree. What do you want to do?" You may be given an abdominal x-ray with a stone in the right lower quadrant or air in the biliary tree.

How to Answer?

Take history and physical examination while resuscitating the patient.

L. Szczurek, D.O., F.A.C.O.S. (✉)
General Surgery Department, Kennedy Health System,
2201 Chapel Avenue West, Suite 100, Cherry Hill, NJ 08002, USA
e-mail: lszczurek@hotmail.com

M.A. Neff, M.D., F.A.C.S.
Minimally Invasive, 2201 Chapel Avenue West, Suite 100,
Cherry Hill, NJ 08002, USA
e-mail: mneffyhs@aol.com

History
  Prior surgery
  Malignancy history
  Overall medical condition
  History suggestive of gallbladder disease
  History of intermittent obstruction classic
Physical Examination
  Vital signs (patient may be unstable)
  Check for surgical scars
  Check for hernias!
Diagnostic Tests
  Full laboratory panel (including liver function tests [LFTs]—may be other stones)
  Obstruction series—air/fluid levels, dilated loops small bowel, ± gallstone
  Computed tomography (CT) scan (not usually necessary)—in addition to the above seen on the obstruction series, you can also see pneumobilia

Surgical Treatment

Resuscitate the patient, including nasogastric tube and intravenous fluids (IVF), then transfer to the operating room(OR) for exploration:
  Full exploratory laparotomy (be prepared to describe this)
  Check the status of the right upper quadrant (RUQ; extensive scarring prevents definitive procedure)
  Longitudinal enterotomy along the antimesenteric border a few centimeters proximal to the stone
  "Milk" stone back gently
  Close enterotomy in two layers
  Check the rest of the intestine for additional stones (~10 %)
  Pay attention to the RUQ (mortality is less in retrospective series if done in separate procedures!)
    Take down fistula and close the bowel in two layers

Cholecystectomy and cholangiogram to look for other stones

(only if inflammation is not severe, patient is stable, and scarring will preclude safe dissection)

Common Curveballs

Patient has history of malignancy

Patient has an associated intra-abdominal process

Patient has severe scarring in RUQ precluding definitive procedure

Patient has postoperative bowel obstruction (missed a second stone)

Patient is septic/unstable

Stone erodes through the hepatic flexure of the colon rather than the duodenum

Examiner asks how to close the fistula

Gallbladder is cancerous, which led to the perforation

Patient develops cholangitis or intra-abdominal abscess postoperative (scenario switch)

Postoperative biliary leak (scenario switch)

Clean Kills

Not checking for hernias

Not getting obstruction series but skipping to CT scan

Not checking for prior surgeries

Not recognizing the problem

Not "milking" back the stone

Performing takedown of fistula in an unstable patient

Summary

Gallstone ileus is a misnomer for a cholecystoenteric fistula in which the gallstone erodes through the gallbladder into the small intestine and causes a mechanical small bowel obstruction. The patient will usually present with the classic signs and symptoms of a small bowel obstruction, including abdominal pain, distention, and nausea and vomiting. The patient may also have a history suggestive of gallbladder disease. A careful abdominal examination should be done to rule out any previous surgical scars or hernias. Obstruction series will show classic signs of an obstruction and possibly the stone and CT scan will show pneumobilia. The surgical treatment is exploratory laparotomy with removal of the obstructing stone. The bowel should be run to make sure that there are no other stones. Take down of the fistula is not required, especially during the first procedure, and is reserved for stable, healthy, young patients with minimal inflammation.

Liver Abscess

Concept

Liver abscess is usually a complication of an underlying disease process (appendicitis, biliary disease, diverticulitis). It is less likely the result of an amebic infection. More commonly today, it is associated with immunosuppression (human immunodeficiency virus [HIV]) or intravenous drug use (IVDU, endocarditis).

Way Question May Be Asked?

"A 35 year-old man is evaluated in the ED for fever, chills, and a constant dull ache in the right flank. He has a history of IVDU, and his CT scan shows multiple liver abscesses. What do you want to do?"

How to Answer?

Take a full history and physical examination.

History
   IVDU
   HIV
   Recent abdominal infections
   Travel history
   History of malignancy (could this be a presentation of metastatic disease?)

Physical Examination
   Full physical, especially abdominal exam (liver enlargement,tenderness)
   Lymphadenopathy

Diagnostic Tests
   Hepatitis panel/LFTs (still working up RUQ pain)
   Complete blood count (CBC)
   Ultrasound of RUQ
   CT scan of the abdomen/pelvis
   Agglutination/compliment fixation tests to rule out an amebic abscess

Surgical Treatment

For an amebic abscess (*Entamoeba histolytica*), administer metronidazole unless there is:
   Secondary infection
   Rupture into biliary tree or abdominal cavity
   Failure to initially improve on antibiotics (may need to be on antibiotics for months if initial improvement is seen)

Pyogenic abscess

Either from biliary tree, portal venous system, or direct extension from adjacent organ

Perform percutaneous drainage and intravenous (IV) antibiotics (can try to treat multiple small abscesses with IV antibiotics)

Use open drainage if percutaneous drainage is not a possibility, which depends on the location of abscess:

Posteriorly through the bed of the 12th rib and extra-peritoneal approach

Interiorly through subcostal incision and extraperitoneal approach

Transperitoneally

Common Curveballs

Patient has history of malignancy

Patient has associated intra-abdominal process

Patient has history of IVDU/HIV

Patient has amebic abscess

Patient has multiple abscesses

You need to perform open drainage and are asked to describe your approach

Amebic abscess ruptures into the abdominal cavity or biliary tree

Examiner asks you to describe treatment of diverticulitis or cholangitis (scenario switch!)

Clean Kills

Not checking for pyogenic abscess from the abdominal source

Not ruling out an amebic abscess

Not getting a biopsy of the abscess wall to rule out malignancy

Mixing up treatment of ecchinococcccal cysts and amebic abscess (ecchinococcccal/hydatid cysts are identified by electrophoresis for ecchinococcus and initially treated with mebendazole; failure to resolve demands first endoscopic retrograde cholangiopancreatography [ERCP] to rule out communication with the biliary tree, then surgery and injection of the cyst with hypertonic saline, avoiding any spillage—anaphylaxis—and performing pericystectomy)

Liver Mass

Concept

Liver mass is usually found during an exploratory laparotomy performed for colon cancer, lower gastrointestinal (GI) bleeding, or other unrelated reasons. It may also be diagnosed incidentally on CT or ultrasound performed on a patient with abdominal pain. Make sure to differentiate solid from cystic lesions here. Hemangioma is the most common benign tumor. Half of adenomas present with spontaneous bleeding.

Way Question May Be Asked?

"A 37-year-old woman is evaluated in the ED for abdominal pain. The CT scan shows a 3-cm mass deep in the right lobe of the liver. What do you want to do?" You may be presented with the scenario of doing an exploratory laparotomy and finding an incidental lesion in the periphery of the liver, or the patient may present as hypotensive with abdominal pain.

How to Answer?

History

Hepatitis

Previous malignancy

Oral contraceptive pill use

Weight loss/anorexia

Race (African and Southeast Asian descent is associated with hepatocellular carcinoma [HCC])

Abdominal pain

Physical Examination

Full physical examination, especially an abdominal examination (liver enlargement, tenderness)

Diagnostic Tests

Hepatitis panel/LFTs

± Alpha fetoprotein (AFP) (if you suspect HCC)

± Carcinoembryonic antigen (CEA) (if you suspect colorectal recurrence)

CBC

Ultrasound of RUQ (used to rule out cyst/abscess—scenario switch)

CT scan of the abdomen/pelvis to characterize the solid nature of the lesion (central scar is associated with focal nodular hyperplasia [FNH])

Magnetic resonance imaging (MRI)

± Tagged red blood cell (RBC) technetium scan (to rule out hemangioma)

± Angiography—may be helpful in evaluating primary malignancies

Differential Diagnosis

Hemangioma

FNH

Adenoma

Malignancy (primary or metastatic)

Surgical Treatment

1. Fine needle aspiration (FNA) under CT guidance—helpful if it diagnoses malignancy, but do not perform if you suspect hepatocellular cancer (elevated AFP, hepatitis B positive, cirrhosis)
2. If FNA is performed, you need a core needle biopsy by laparoscopy or open surgery
3. Treatment
   (a) FNH—observation unless becomes patient becomes symptomatic
   (b) Adenoma—stop birth control pills (BCP) and observe for 6 months; resect if:
       Patient becomes symptomatic
       Adenoma increases in size during the observation period
       Patient intends on becoming pregnant
   (c) Malignancy—
       can resect metastatic disease if it is a colon or neuroendocrine malignancy, as long as primary site is controlled
       (5-year survival is ~30% from metastectomy for colorectal cancer if <5 metastases and less than 5 cm in size)
       For hepatocellular carcinoma, be prepared to describe liver resection
   (d) Hemangioma—diagnosis is made by CT, MRI, or tagged RBC scan
       Observe unless very large or symptomatic
       Can cause pain, hemolysis, and congestive heart failure
       Spontaneous rupture is rare (1–2%)
       Embolization is the first choice if patient is symptomatic
       Often surgically treated by enucleation
4. Incidental liver lesion
   Biopsy is necessary
   Perform FNA to make sure it is not cystic or hemangioma
   Consider intraoperative ultrasound
   You can perform a wedge resection if lesion is small and peripheral

Common Curveballs

Patient has a history of malignancy
Examiner asks when you will perform resection for metastatic disease
Liver nodule is found during exploratory laparotomy and you are asked what would you do
Patient has cystic lesion in the liver (scenario switch)

Adenoma/hemangioma bleeds spontaneously during your observation period and patient presents in hemorrhagic shock
FNA is negative

Clean Kills

Not ruling out a cystic lesion
Not knowing treatment for FNH or hepatoma
Sticking a needle into a hemangioma
Not knowing how to describe your liver resection
Not trying to biopsy a liver lesion found during an exploratory laparotomy
Not performing the CT scan with contrast
Performing metastatectomy for breast or stomach cancer
Performing an FNA on hepatocellular cancer
Performing a liver resection laparoscopically
Getting lost in a discussion about angiographic embolization when the patient clearly needs to go to the OR (resuscitate/check coagulation first)

Choledocholithiasis

Concept

Common bile duct stones can be primary (formed in the common bile duct) or secondary (passed from the gallbladder into the common bile duct). Many common duct stones are asymptomatic, but the presentation can range from biliary colic to cholangitis. Approximately 1–2 % of patients will have a retained common duct stone after laparoscopic cholecystectomy.

Way Question May Be Asked?

"A 65-year-old woman presents to the ER with a complaint of some mild right upper quadrant abdominal pain that has been going on for the past few days. The pain is worse after eating and she has had some nausea but no vomiting. She was bought to the ER by her daughter, who came to visit today and was concerned that her mother's skin looked yellow. What do you want to do?"

How to Answer?

History
   Medical history

Surgical history

Social history (especially alcohol use)

History of any cancer in patient or family

Detailed questions regarding symptoms

Physical Examination

Vital signs

General—jaundice, diaphoresis, metal status

Abdominal—right upper quadrant pain, Murphy's sign

Chartcot's triad—RUQ pain, fever, jaundice

Reynold's pentad—the above triad plus hypotension and change in mental status

Diagnostic Tests

Full laboratory panel including LFTs, amylase, and lipase—expect elevated transaminases and direct bilirubin, possible elevated white blood cells (WBCs)

RUQ ultrasound—gallstones, wall thickness, ± pericholecystic fluid, dilated common bile duct [CBD], possible stone in duct

Magnetic resonance cholangiopancreatography—diagnostic for evaluating stones in the common bile duct

ERCP—diagnostic and therapeutic; you can identify and remove stones in the common bile duct as well as perform a sphincterotomy and place a stent if needed

Percutaneous transhepatic cholangiography (PTC)—also diagnostic and therapeutic for identifying and removing stones

Surgical Treatment

First ensure nothing by mouth (NPO) and administer IVF and IV antibiotics.

The patient should undergo ERCP with removal of the stones and decompression of the common bile duct, followed by laparoscopic (possible open) cholecystectomy, which was described in the previous chapter.

If ERCP is unavailable, the patient will need an intraoperative cholangiogram and stone removal; this may be done laparoscopically or open.

Laparoscopic intraoperative cholangiogram can be done via the cystic duct or using stay sutures and a choledochotomy. The cholangiogram is taken and stones are identified. The scope is fed down the duct and the stones are removed with the wire basket or snare. You can also try a Fogarty catheter. Performing the cholangiogram via the cystic duct limits the size of the stones that can be removed, but it is much easier technically because it avoids laparoscopic suturing of the duct.

In an open intraoperative cholangiogram, stay sutures are placed in the duct, a choledochotomy is made, the cholangiogram is taken, and the stones are identified. The stones are removed and the duct closed around a T-tube.

If you are unable to remove the stones due to impaction, you can perform a choledochoduodenotomy or a Roux-en-Y hepaticojejunostomy.

If a stone is impacted at the ampulla and cannot be removed via choledochotomy, perform a transduodenalsphincteroplasty with an incision at 11 o'clock.

Common Curveballs

You do not have ERCP available

You are not able to get the stones out of the common duct

The stone is impacted at the ampulla

Patient returns after surgery with similar symptoms (retained stone)

Patient has a bile leak around the T-tube

The T-tube gets dislodged postoperatively

Clean Kills

Missing choledocholithiasis

Not knowing what to do if you do not have access to ERCP

Not knowing the general steps to intraoperative cholangiogram (if you cannot perform a laparoscopic CBD exploration, it is always acceptable to convert to an open procedure)

Missing a retained stone postoperatively

Not doing a final intraopcholangiogram

Not leaving a T-tube

Not knowing proper management of the T-tube

Summary

Choledocholithiasis is a common surgical issue encountered by the general surgeon. Patients often present with similar symptoms as those with biliary colic or cholecystitis, but during their workup they are found to have an elevated direct bilirubin or a dilated common bile duct on radiology studies. Once this is identified, choledocholithiasis must be excluded prior to cholecystectomy. This workup may include further radiology studies such as MRCP, ERCP, or an intraoperative cholangiogram. The ultimate surgical treatment is removal of both the common duct stones and the gallbladder.

Choledochal Cyst

Concept

This congenital cystic disease of the biliary tract can be associated with other anomalies, such as intestinal atresia, imperforate anus, and pancreatic divism. Most importantly, choledochal cysts are considered to be premalignant lesions:

Type 1: Fusiform dilatation of entire CBD
Type 2: True diverticulum off the CBD
Type 3: Dilatation of the distal CDB involving the sphincter of Oddi
Type 4: Multiple intrahepatic and extrahepatic cysts
Type 5: Intrahepatic cysts only

Way the Question May Be Asked?

"A 10-year-old child is brought to the ED by her parents with a complaint of right upper abdominal pain, nausea, and a fever. Her parents note that the whites of her eyes have turned yellow over the past few days. What do you want to do?"

You may also be given a similar scenario of a younger child with similar symptoms and a palpable right upper abdominal mass on examination.

How to Answer?

History
　Complete medical history, including any anomalies noted at birth
　Careful questioning of patient and parents with regards to history and presentation of symptoms (differentiate between simple biliary colic)
Physical Examination
　Vital signs—fever is common
　Signs of jaundice: scleral icterus, yellowing of skin
　Complete abdominal examination—check for a pain or a palpable mass in the RUQ
Diagnostic Tests
　Full laboratory panel, including LFTs, which will often show an elevated bilirubin consistent with the obstructive jaundice
　RUQ ultrasound—cystic mass that is separate from the gallbladder
　HIDA scan—filling of the cyst followed by delayed emptying
　CT scan—useful for evaluating the intrahepatic, distal CBD and pancreatic anatomy

　MRCP—criterion standard for evaluating the ducts for choledochal cysts
　ERCP—invasive and has a high rate of pancreatitis and cholangitis with choledochal cysts

Surgical Treatment

For all types, the treatment is resection of the entire involved area due to the risk of malignancy.

Type 1—resection of cyst and hepaticojejunostomy: The gallbladder dissected out and clipped at cystic artery. The hepatic duct is identified and divided above the cyst. The cyst is dissected off and removed en bloc with the gallbladder. A standard 40-cm retrocolic Roux limb is created and anastomosed to the hepatic duct in an end-to-side fashion using absorbable monofilament suture.
Type 2—primary resection off the CBD
Type 3—resection with choledochojejunostomy or marsupialization of the cyst, usually through a transduodenal approach
Type 4—resection, may need liver lobectomy
Type 5—resection, may need liver lobectomy or transplant

Common Curveballs

Patient is an adult and the cyst was missed as a child (can be confused with other biliary pathology, such as cholecystitis or choledocholithiasis)
Examiner asks about the complications of the procedure (stricture is most common)
Remember that type 1 is the most common type.

Clean Kills

Not removing the cyst (it has malignant potential)
Performing an ERCP (it has a high rate of cholangitis and pancreatitis)
Missing the diagnosis (can have a similar presentation as cholecystitis/choledocholithiasis but is more common in children)
Not ruling out other anomalies in a newborn

Summary

Choledochal cysts are congenital cysts of the biliary tract that are thought to be caused by reflux of pancreatic

enzymes during development. There are five types of choledochal cysts based on location, with type 1 being the most common. Patients usually present before the age of 10 years with a combination of fever, jaundice, and a palpable right upper quadrant mass. Laboratory studies will usually show elevated direct bilirubin, which is consistent with the obstructive jaundice. The best test for the overall evaluation of the bile ducts is an MRCP. The definitive treatment is complete surgical resection of the area involving the cyst.

Hepatobiliary—Cholecystitis

Concept

The majority of gallstones are asymptomatic and are found on imaging studies that were performed for other reasons. To become symptomatic, the stones must block the cystic duct. Formation of gallstones involves four factors: supersaturation of secreted bile, concentration of bile within the gallbladder, crystal nucleation, and gallbladder dysmotility. They can present as anywhere along the spectrum; biliary colic, chronic cholecystitis, or acute cholecystitis.

Way Question May Be Asked?

"A 40-year-old woman presents to the ED with a complaint of right upper quadrant pain radiating to her upper back associated with nausea and vomiting. The pain started after she ate pizza for dinner and has not improved. She has had similar episodes in the past but the pain would only last a short time and go away. What do you want to do?" You may be given RUQ ultrasound results that show a gallstone in the neck of the gallbladder and laboratory tests with a mildly elevated WBC and transaminases.

How to Answer?

History
   The classic Fs: fat, fertile, forty, female (gallbladder disease is more common in this population)
   Medical history
   Surgical history
   Last menstrual period (for females)
   History suggestive of gallbladder disease (RUQ pain after eating fatty foods)
Physical Examination
   Vital signs
   Complete abdominal examination, including Murphy's sign
   Diagnostic Tests

Full set of laboratory tests, including CBC, basic metabolic panel, LFTs, amylase, lipase, and pregnancy test for females
RUQ ultrasound: look for stones, wall thickening, pericholecystic fluid, size of the common bile duct
As long as the common bile duct is normal size on ultrasound and the bilirubin is within normal limits on laboratory studies, no other studies should be needed.
HIDA scan—can be used to rule out acute cholecystitis in situations in which the patient is risk or has concurrent medical issues that prevent the patient from going to the OR at the present time or to rule out acalculouscholecystitis

Surgical Treatment

Administer NPO, IVF, and IV antibiotics
OR for laparoscopic (possible open) cholecystectomy
Laparoscopic cholecystectomy: Use a 5-mm periumbilical port, 10–12 mm subxyphoid port, and 2, 0.5-mm RUQ ports. The peritoneum is dissected off the infundibulum of the gallbladder to expose the triangle of Calot, including the cystic duct and artery. The cystic duct should be visualized, going directly from the gallbladder to the common bile duct. A window is created behind the cystic duct and the artery. Clips are placed on either side of each structure and the duct and artery are transected between the clips. The remainder of the adhesions of the gallbladder to the liver bed are taken down using electrocautery. Once the gallbladder is freed, it is placed into an endobag and removed from the abdomen through the subxyphoid port. The gallbladder fossa is then inspected and hemostasis is achieved. The fascia of the subxyphoid port site is closed along with the skin.

Open cholecystectomy: Make a RUQ Kocher incision two finger breaths below the right costal margin. The gallbladder is grasped with two clamps. The same dissection as described in the laparoscopic section above is followed. The duct and artery may be clipped or tied off using silk suture. The gallbladder is then removed from the fossa, also using electrocautery. Hemostasis is achieved and the incision closed.

If needed, both procedures may be performed with an intraoperative cholangiogram.

If the patient is too unstable due to other medical conditions to undergo surgery, intervention radiology can be consulted for placement of a percutaneous cholecystostomy tube.

Common Curveballs

Patient has had a myocardial infarction or other problem on admission that makes them high risk or unstable for the OR (what do you do?)

Patient has the signs and symptoms of cholecystitis but no stones on the RUQ ultrasound (possible acalculous cholecystitis; suspect this in an intensive care unit patient and check the HIDA scan)

Patient has a dilated common bile duct

Patient has elevated bilirubin

Patient has a postoperative bile leak (check a HIDA scan, interventional radiology (IR) consult for drain and ERCP for stent)

Gallbladder is necrotic and falls apart during your laparoscopic dissection

Bile is seen in liver bed when inspecting for hemostasis

Clean Kills

Missing a possible choledocholithiasis

Missing a postoperative bile leak

Ordering HIDA scans with ejection fractions

Not doing a cholangiogram when you are unsure of the anatomy

Performing subtotal cholecystectomy laparoscopically

Summary

The majority of gallstones are asymptomatic and are found incidentally on other studies. Gallbladder disease usually presents as episodes of right upper quadrant pain radiating to the upper back, often associated with nausea or vomiting. The episodes are frequently brought on by fatty foods. The patient may have an elevated WBC and transaminases. Right upper quadrant ultrasound is the criterion standard test for evaluation of the gallbladder. The surgical treatment is laparoscopic (possible open) cholecystectomy.

Postcholecystectomy Cholangitis

Concept

In questions on postcholecystectomy cholangitis, the suggestion is that a stone was missed and the patient returns with an obstructed biliary tree and is septic from ascending cholangitis. Prompt treatment is important here, as well as stabilizing patient in the intensive care unit (ICU) setting.

Way Question May Be Asked?

"A 55-year-old man is seen in the ER 1 year after a laparoscopic cholecystectomy with fever, chills, RUQ pain, and jaundice. What do you want to do?"

The interval after laparoscopic cholecystectomy may vary. Your differential diagnosis needs to include retained stone, new stone, stricture, tumor, and extrinsic compression.

How to Answer?

Start with the ABCs here because patient is septic from cholangitis. Obtain any relevant history and physical examination while resuscitating the patient.

History

    Time course

    History of hepatitis

    History of hemolysis

    Malignancies

    Previous operative indications/report

Physical

    Abdominal examination

    Confirm jaundice

Diagnostic Tests

    Full laboratory panel, including LFTs

    Plain x-rays of abdomen

    RUQ ultrasound (look for dilated ducts, evaluate CBD, see mass?)

Surgical Treatment

1. ABCs
2. IVF resuscitation
3. ICU
4. Central venous pressure line
5. Antibiotics (broad spectrum)
6. Ultrasound of RUQ
7. ERCP to drain CBD and remove stone if possible (needs to be under 1.5 cm in size); biopsy any mass
8. PTC if ERCP fails to drain biliary tree
9. Surgery if ERCP/PTC both fail after your best attempts to stabilize the patient

    The goal here is to drain the biliary tree by whatever means possible.

    (a) CBD exploration: Extract any stone. If you cannot, place a T-tube and close. Remember to:

        Always do intra-operative cholangiogram (IOC) when placing a T-tube and use absorbable sutures in CBD closure

        Use a choledochoscope, biliary fogarties, irrigation, and Stone forceps

        Bring out T-tube through abdominal wall with as straight a course as possible

    (b) Other options include the following:

        Choledochoduodenostomy (and leave stone behind)

        Sphincteroplasty (description below)

        Choledochojejunostomy

Common Curveballs

Porta hepatic is severely scarred down and you cannot safely mobilize the duodenum

Gastroenterologist is not available for ERCP

Stone cannot be removed by ERCP

PTC does not work to decompress biliary system

Patient has an iatrogenic injury to CBD (scenario switch)

Examiner asks you to describe transduodenal sphincteroplasty (open duodenum longitudinally, open medial wall of ampulla directly onto stone itself, identify pancreatic duct orifice [may need to give IV glucagon here], suture ductal mucosa to duodenal mucosa with fine absorbable suture)

Patient has a malignancy

Patient has a stricture

Patient has other comorbidities (recent myocardial infarction or acute respiratory failure; scenario changes to ICU management)

Clean Kills

Not trying ERCP or PTC but rushing to surgery

Not knowing other options besides CBD exploration and placing T-tube

Not being able to describe CBD exploration

Trying to perform anything laparoscopically

Not stabilizing patient prior to any maneuvers

Discussing endoscopic lithotripsy

Remember the indications for CBD exploration:

Positive intraoperative cholangiogram

Large stone

Impacted stone (usually distally impacted)

Multiple stones

Cholangitis and failed ERCP/PTC

Postcholecystectomy Jaundice

Concept

You may be faced with a variety of postcholecystectomy problems. Always be methodical in your workup of these patients and do not rush to the OR.

Way Question May Be Asked?

"A patient returns to your office 1 week after an uneventful laparoscopic cholecystectomy performed by your partner for symptomatic cholelithiasis and is jaundiced. What do you want to do?"

The scenario may happen more immediately after surgery. You may be given a difficult intraoperative dissection or a history of CBD stones.

How to Answer?

History
  Hepatitis
  Hemolysis
  Indications for surgery
  Operative report (was IOC performed?)
  Timing of jaundice
  Color change of urine/stool
  Signs or symptoms of cholangitis
Physical Examination
  Check for icterus
  Check incisions
  Full abdominal examination
Diagnostic Testing
  General laboratory panels, especially LFTs and amylase
  Abdominal x-rays
  Ultrasound of RUQ (biliary tree dilation, stones, biloma, extrinsic compression?)
  Hepatobiliary scan (look for CBD occlusion or leak, look for cystic duct/duct of Lushka leak)
  CT scan (look for biloma, extrinsic compression of biliary tree)
  Drain percutaneously

Surgical Treatment

Admit to hospital

Start antibiotics

Get appropriate studies as above

Surgical management based on HIDA/ERCP findings

1. CBD leak
   Stent across with ERCP
   Drain biloma percutaneously
2. Cystic duct leak
   Stent across with ERCP
   Drain biloma percutaneously
   All will close if there is no distal obstruction
3. CBD occlusion
   Perform ERCP to determine nature of obstruction, retrieve stone, sphincterotomy
   If iatrogenic, schedule the patient for exploration (wait 3–6 weeks as long as the patient is not septic) for clip removal, repair of CBD over T-tube, or choledochojejunostomy
4. Duct of Lushka leak
   Drain biloma

      Ensure no distal obstruction

      Patient may need to return to OR to suture/ligate

5. If creating a choledochojejunostomy, use a Roux limb, end to side, with end of jejunum against the abdominal wall so you have some access to the biliary tree if need be

6. Do not forget the other options that are appropriate in certain scenarios:

      Hepaticojejunostomy

      Choledochoduodenostomy

Common Curveballs

ERCP is not available (do not forget about PTC)

Patient develops cholangitis

Examiner ask how you will discuss an iatrogenic injury with your patient

Examiner asks how to treat injury to CBD (can repair primarily if <50 % over T-tube)

Examiner asks how to treat retained stone that fails ERCP (describe CBD exploration, scenario switch)

Examiner asks how to construct choledochojejunostomy

There is not enough length to perform primary repair to the CBD

Simple drainage of biloma does not work

Electrolyte abnormalities occur from high drain output

Clean Kills

Rushing back in to reoperate

Not getting ultrasound, HIDA scan, or ERCP

Not knowing ways to treat CBD leak or occlusion

Not recognizing possible iatrogenic injury to the CBD

Not being honest with your patient about an injury when the examiner asks the ethical question of how you discuss the situation with your patient

Pancreas

Linda Szczurek, Jonathan Nguyen, and Marc A. Neff

Acute Pancreatitis

Concept

This life-threatening condition represents a massive retroperitoneal burn with tremendous amounts of third spacing. It may be secondary to alcoholism, gallstones (most common in the United States), tumor, elevated triglycerides, medication, post-endoscopic retrograde cholangiopancreatography (ERCP), pancreatic divism, or even perforated ulcer. Approximately 80–90 % of the episodes are self-limiting; the remainder of cases progress to release a massive inflammatory response.

Way Question May Be Asked?

"You are called down to the emergency room (ER) to evaluate a patient with severe epigastric pain, vomiting, and history of recent alcohol use. What do you want to do?"

You may or may not be given history of gallstones or alcohol use. The patient may have elevated amylase. You need to rule out other causes of severe epigastric abdominal pain, including gastritis, perforated ulcer, rupture of esopha-

L. Szczurek, D.O., F.A.C.O.S. (✉)
General Surgery Department, Kennedy Health System,
2201 Chapel Avenue West, Suite 100, Cherry Hill, NJ 08002, USA
e-mail: lszczurek@hotmail.com

J. Nguyen, D.O.
General Surgery, University of Medicine & Dentistry
of New Jersey, Stratford, NJ, USA
e-mail: diligenceb@yahoo.com

M.A. Neff, M.D., F.A.C.S.
Minimally Invasive, 2201 Chapel Avenue West, Suite 100,
Cherry Hill, NJ 08002, USA
e-mail: mneffyhs@aol.com

gus (if there is history of emesis), abdominal aortic aneurysm (AAA), ischemia, and gastric volvulus.

How to Answer?

Key parts of the answer include assessment of severity, determination of etiology, aggressive volume resuscitation, appropriate support (nutrition/ventilator), operative intervention when appropriate, and recognition of complications.

History
  Gallstones
  Alcohol use
  Recent new medications
  Timing of pain with retching/vomiting
  History of peptic ulcer disease/AAA
Physical Examination
  Perform a complete physical examination, including the following:
    Vital signs (tachycardia/hypotension)
    Crepitus over chest/neck (to rule out Boerhaave's syndrome)
    Abdominal examination (peritonitis, Grey-Turner's sign—flank ecchymosis, Cullen's sign—periumbilical ecchymosis, both are indications of hemorrhagic pancreatitis)
    Prior incisions
    Hernias (could this be simply obstruction?)
Diagnostic Tests
  Complete laboratory panel, including amylase, lipase, calcium, albumin, lactate dehydrogenase (LDH), arterial blood gas (depending on severity of illness)
  Chest x-ray (CXR; to rule out esophageal rupture)
  Abdominal x-ray (AXR; to look for ileus, sentinel loop, obstruction, aortic calcifications, free air, and gallstones)
  Ultrasound (to look for gallstones, ductal dilatation, examine pancreas, and rule out AAA)

M.A. Neff (ed.), *Passing the General Surgery Oral Board Exam*,
DOI 10.1007/978-1-4614-7663-4_9, © Springer Science+Business Media New York 2014

Computed tomography (CT) scan (to look for pancreatic inflammation; there is also a staging mortality predictor based on CT findings)

Ranson's Criteria

On admission: age >55 years

White blood cells (WBC) >16,000 cell/mm³

Glucose >200 mg/dL

Serum glutamic oxaloacetic transaminase >250 IU/L

LDH >350 IU/L

During first 48 h: Hematocrit falls by 10 %

Blood urea nitrogen rises by 5 mg/dL

Calcium <8 mg/dL

Fluid sequestration >6 L

PO$_2$ <60 mmHg

Ranson's score greater than or equal to 3 indicates severe pancreatitis

Surgical Treatment

1. Supportive care with intravenous fluids, nothing by mouth (NPO), nasogastric tube, serial laboratory panels, H2 blockers, intravenous (IV) analgesics
2. CT scan to evaluate for complications and necrosis
3. Ventilatory/nutritional support where appropriate (patient will likely deteriorate and will need transfer to the intensive care unit, central venous pressure line, intubation, and total parenteral nutrition [TPN])
4. Most patients should improve in next several days (your patient, of course, will not!)
5. If patient fails to improve, check repeat CT.
    (a) Perform fine needle aspiration (FNA) if any necrosis is present and patient has a fever of unknown origin (can observe sterile necrosis)
    (b) If FNA is positive, then perform a <u>necrosectomy</u>:
        If cultures/gram stain are positive or patient has a gross infection, administer IV antibiotics.
        Make a Chevron incision.
        Open up the lesser sac.
        Debride all devitalized necrotic tissues.
        Perform a large-volume lavage of the abdomen.
        Leave large drains in the lesser sac.
        Perform a jejunostomy.
6. Patient develops an epigastric mass:
    (a) Obtain CT or ultrasound to confirm <u>pseudocyst.</u>
    (b) Do not do an FNA.
    (c) ± ERCP to rule out ductal communication.
    (d) Feed past ampulla or TPN for 8 weeks and reassess (allow wall to mature).
    (e) There are various options for internal drainage depending on location.

7. Patient gets better and cause was gallstones
    (a) You need ERCP preoperatively if choldecholithiasis is suspected—possible sphincterotomy and stone retrieval.
    (b) Be prepared for an intraoperative cholangiogram and common bile duct exploration.
    (c) Perform a laparoscopic cholecystectomy during the same admission.

Common Curveballs

Patient develops pancreatic necrosis

Patient develops a pseudocyst

Patient develops pancreatic ascites

Patient develops ascending cholangitis (scenario switch to a discussion of how to drain a dilated biliary tree)

Patient is pregnant

Patient has gallstone pancreatitis

Patient later presents with symptoms of chronic pancreatitis

Patient develops upper gastrointestinal (GI) bleeding related to splenic vein thrombosis

Examiner asks you to discuss the use of antibiotics/somatostatin

Examiner asks you to discuss Ranson's criteria

Patient has an obstructing tumor/gallstone as the cause for pancreatitis

Patient needs nutritional/respiratory support and asks you to discuss these modalities

Patient develops delirium tremens (DTs) as result of alcohol withdrawal

Clean Kills

Trying to percutaneously drain infected necrosis

Not recognizing/appropriately treating the complications of pancreatitis

Failing to rule out other possible causes of severe epigastric/abdominal pain

Trying to do anything but cholecystectomy laparoscopically

Not being aggressive in your supportive care for the patient

Not trying to identify the etiology of the pancreatitis

Not performing intra-operative cholangiogram (IOC) when doing a laparoscopic cholecystectomy after a bout of pancreatitis

Summary

Acute pancreatitis can present along a very wide spectrum from mild to life threatening. The two most

common causes of acute pancreatitis in the United States are gallstones and alcohol use. Patients usually have a complaint of severe epigastric pain radiating to the back, often associated with nausea and vomiting. The diagnosis is confirmed by elevated amylase and lipase on laboratory studies. After the diagnosis is made, the cause of the pancreatitis should be identified. Most patients will respond to conservative management with NPO, fluids, and pain control followed by cholecystectomy after resolution of the pancreatitis if the cause is gallstones. However, some patients will progress to either necrotizing pancreatitis or develop a pseudocyst and may need surgical intervention.

Chronic Pancreatitis

Concept

The etiology of chronic pancreatitis includes alcohol abuse, hyperparathyroidism, cystic fibrosis, pancreatic divism, and trauma. Alcohol-related chronic pancreatitis is most common in developed countries. There are a variety of suggested mechanisms, including hypersecretion of protein from acinar cells, plugging of pancreatic ducts with protein precipitates, and pancreatic ductal hypertension. Pathology includes acinar loss, glandular shrinkage, proliferative fibrosis, calcification, and ductal stricturing.

Way Question May Be Asked?

"A 45-year-old alcoholic with a history of several episodes of pancreatitis presents now with worsening abdominal pain and is taking narcotics around the clock. What do you want to do?"

You could be presented with any of the complications of chronic pancreatitis. Be careful to rule out other complications of pancreatitis (ascites, pseudocyst, acute pancreatitis) before diving into discussion of the management of chronic pancreatitis.

How to Answer?

History
  Abdominal pain (epigastric, radiation to back, continuous or relapsing)
  Anorexia
  Weight loss
  Diabetes mellitus type 1 (~33 % of patients)
  Steatorrhea (~25 % of patients)

  Classic Tetrad: abdominal pain, weight loss, diabetes mellitus, and steatorrhea
  Narcotic use
  Flares of pancreatitis
  Etiology of pancreatitis
Physical Examination
  Palpable mass (pseudocyst)
  Stigmata of alcoholic liver disease
  Abdominal examination (ascites and epigastric tenderness are consistent with acute pancreatitis)
Diagnostic Studies
  Laboratory tests (only for completeness—IV secretin and cholecystokinin stimulation with collection of pancreatic effluent, 72-h fecal fat, glucose tolerance testing to measure endocrine function)
  AXR (pancreatic calcifications are 95 % specific if seen)
  CT (evaluate parenchymal disease, pseudocyst, ductal dilatation, parenchymalatrophy, or irregular contour)
  Magnetic resonance cholangiopancreatography (MRCP; evaluate ductal anatomy for stricture or disruption)
  ERCP (ductal dilatation, strictures, calculi, *chain of lakes* pancreatogram)

Surgical Treatment

1. Nonoperative therapy (symptomatic treatment)
   (a) Control abdominal pain: abstinence from alcohol, dietary manipulation (low-fat, small-volume meals), and nonnarcotic analgesics first (often failure of this is an indication for surgery)
   (b) Treatment for endocrine insufficiency: use exogenous insulin carefully (hypoglycemia can arise as a result of poor nutrient absorption)
   (c) Treatment for exocrine insufficiency: low-fat diet, exogenous pancreatic enzymes
       If medical therapy fails (which of course it will!):
       If there is a stricture/obstruction of the duct, you need to rule out cancer, which includes a thorough workup with CT, MRCP, and endoscopic ultrasound (EUS). If all of these are negative, then you can manage with ERCP and a stent.
       Indications for surgery include intractable pain, biliary/pancreatic duct or duodenal obstruction, pseudocyst, pseudoanuerysm, and the inability to rule out cancer.
2. What is size of the pancreatic duct?
   (a) Large pancreatic duct → Peustow procedure
       Side-to-side pancreaticojejunostomy with success rates of 60–90 %: The procedure decompresses the entire duct. You need a duct greater than

7 mm in diameter, pancreatic calcifications, and pancreatic-jejunal anastomosis longer than 6 cm. It does not affect endocrine/exocrine insufficiency.

Make a Chevron incision, divide the gastrocolic ligament to enter the lesser sac, expose the entire anterior surface of the pancreas, create a Roux-en-Y, and anastomose to the entire pancreatic duct.

(b) Small pancreatic duct → pancreatic resection

Pylorus-preserving pancreaticoduodenectomy for a patient with chronic pancreatitis: There should be no ductal dilatation and disease should be primarily in the head of the gland. It preserves endocrine function in the body/tail.

3. Ampullary stenosis→

(a) Ampullary procedures: Transduodenal sphincteroplasty is helpful if there is focal obstruction at the ampullary orifice in a patient with pancreatic divisum and stenosis of minor pancreatic duct papilla (these procedures have generally fallen out of favor)

4. Celiac block can be considered for patients who fail operative interventions.

Common Curveballs

Patient presents with a complication of chronic pancreatitis:
Pain
Pseudoaneurysm
Splenic vein thrombosis
Obstruction (GI or biliary tract)
Exocrine/endocrine deficiency
Pseudocyst
Patient has an anastomotic leak after Peustow procedure
Examiner asks you to describe the Peustow procedure
Pancreatic duct is "large" initially, then changes to "small"
Patient develops postoperative hepatic failure (alcoholic liver disease)
Patient has DTs postoperatively

Clean Kills

Not getting an ERCP/CT scan
Not knowing what operation to offer for a "large" pancreatic duct
Not knowing the complications of chronic pancreatitis
Not being able to describe the Peustow procedure
Offering the patient a total pancreatectomy or 95 % distal pancreatectomy instead of the more standard options

Summary

In the United States, chronic pancreatitis is most commonly caused by alcohol abuse. Patients present with frequent episodes of epigastric pain, often radiating to the back. They may also have diabetes or steatorrhea that are both caused by "burn out" of the pancreas. A CT scan can be used to evaluate the parenchyma of the pancreas; MRCP and ERCP are best for the ductal anatomy. The primary treatment is nonoperative with supportive care: pain management, insulin, and pancreatic enzymes. If there is any stricture/obstruction, cancer needs to be ruled out. The indications for surgical intervention include intractable pain, biliary/pancreatic duct or duodenal obstruction, pseudocyst/pseudoaneurysm, or if cancer cannot be ruled out. The type of surgical intervention depends on the presence or absence of ductal dilatation and the location of any stricture/obstruction.

Pancreatic Cancer

Concept

Approximately 90 % of patients with pancreatic cancer will be unresectable, with a mean survival time of 3 months. The key is to determine who is a candidate for resection. You will likely be given a patient whom you need to explore to determine resectability.

Way Question May Be Asked?

"A 61-year-old man comes to your office with recent weight loss. A CT scan ordered by his family doctor shows a mass in the head of the pancreas. What do you want to do?"

The question may present as just weight loss or obstructive jaundice, or examiners may be direct and get right into the thick of it.

How to Answer?

Be methodical here!
History
Smoking
Anorexia/weight loss
Alcohol use
Back pain/abdominal pain
Family history of cancer
(Classic is painless jaundice)
Physical Examination
Mass in right upper quadrant (liver or distended nontender gallbladder)

Diagnostic Testing

Full laboratory panel, including liver function tests (LFTs), albumin, Alpha fetoprotein (AFP), CA19-9, and carcinoembryonic antigen (CEA)

Routine preoperative studies (electrocardiogram, CXR)

CT scan—triple phase with thin section through the pancreas (look for metastases, enlarged lymph nodes, or vascular involvement)

ERCP—obtain biopsy/brushings/cytology (stent patient only if there is severe jaundice, unrelenting itching, or abnormal LFTs, especially coagulation)

Angiogram with venous phase (look for encasement of the superior mesenteric artery, superior mesenteric vein [SMV], and portal vein, and rule out replaced right hepatic artery)

EUS—not necessary but can help stage tumor and FNA

Staging laparoscopy for uncertain staging

Do not perform a percutaneous biopsy of a possibly resectable tumor (you risk dissemination along the tract)

Differential Diagnosis

Remember other causes of obstructive jaundice if this is what you are presented with:

Stricture

Stone

Extrinsic compression

Malignancy (duodenal, ampullary, cholangio, pancreatic)

Surgical Treatment

1. Laparoscope patient before you open to look for peritoneal implants
   (a) If found, then perform a biliary and gastric bypass laparoscopically
2. Make a Chevron incision
3. Perform a full abdominal exploration and evaluate for resectability (check for hepatic metastases, lymph node metastases outside of the resection zone, and make liberal use of frozen sections)
   "Clockwise resection"
4. Cattell–Braasch maneuver:
   Ligate the middle colic vein
   Expose the SMV
5. Extended Kocher maneuver:
   Ligate the right gonadal vein
6. Portal dissection:
   Ligate the gastroduodenal artery
   Dissect out the gallbladder
   Transect the common hepatic duct just proximal to the cystic duct
   (Be careful as the hepatic artery can course posterior to the portal vein)
7. Transect the stomach

At the level of the third/fourth transverse vein on the lesser curve and confluence of gastroepiploic veins on greater curve
± Pylorus preserving

8. Transect the jejunum
   10 cm distal to ligament of Treitz
9. Transect the pancreas at the level of the portal vein
   If adherent, use proximal and distal control and resect the anterior wall; repair with vein patch
   Take a frozen section to check pancreatic/biliary margins
10. Vagotomy
    "Counter-clockwise reconstruction"
11. End-to-side pancreaticojejunostomy
    Use two layers over a stent
12. End-to-side choledochojejunostomy
13. End-to-side gastrojejunostomy
    Antecolic in two layers
14. Gastrostomy
15. Jejunostomy
16. Use lots of drains!

Common Curveballs

Replaced right hepatic artery (what is its course?)

Tumor is invading the portal vein (discovered during the course of the operation)

You are not able to determine malignancy even with intraoperative biopsies (will you do a Whipple?)

There are complications of the Whipple procedure

There is a leak at any of the anastomoses

Patient has an abscess

Patient has delayed gastric emptying

Patient has a marginal ulcer

Patient has a pancreatic fistula

Patient has a bile leak

Patient has an intraoperative injury to the middle colic vein

There are peritoneal implants (what type of bypass operation will you perform?)

Tumor is in tail of pancreas (perform distal pancreatectomy)

Patient presents as acute pancreatitis (scenario switch)

Examiner asks you how to determine resectability

Patient is malnourished

Examiner asks when you will place the biliary stent preoperatively

Clean Kills

Not performing adequate staging workup to rule out unresectable disease

Not knowing how to describe a Whipple operation

Not knowing how to describe a bypass operation

Performing a percutaneous biopsy of the pancreatic mass in potentially resectable lesions

Performing a total pancreatectomy

Summary

Pancreatic cancer is usually diagnosed late in its disease course, leading to high mortality rates. Initial workup should also include imaging to determine the depth of invasion and any vascular involvement. The big question is whether the mass is resectable. EUS may be helpful in small or difficult-to-define masses. If there is any uncertainty, perform a laparoscopic staging procedure prior to Whipple. Know how to do a Whipple procedure.

Pancreatic Pseudocyst

Concept

A pancreatic pseudocyst is a walled-off collection of pancreatic enzymes and inflammatory fluid typically in the lesser sac (with the boundaries formed by the lesser sac) or within the pancreas itself that is bounded by a nonepithelialized wall of fibrotic tissue. The patient can develop symptoms related to size (obstruction, pain) or erosion into other structures (bleeding).

Way Question May Be Asked?

"A 48-year-old man with a history of alcohol abuse and pancreatitis presents to the ER with abdominal pain. Workup reveals a 4-cm pancreatic pseudocyst."

The question may be about abdominal pain in a patient with a history of pancreatitis, or you could be given the formation of a pseudocyst after an initial bout of pancreatitis with the patient still in the hospital.

How to Answer?

Complete History and Physical Examination
  Weight loss
  Vomiting
  Abdominal mass
  Trauma
  Alcoholism
  History of acute or chronic pancreatitis
  Palpable mass

Diagnostic Tests
  Appropriate laboratory tests (amylase, WBC)
  Ultrasound (good for screening)
  CT scan (criterion standard)
Be complete, but do not dwell on these because the examiner is trying to get to your management here.
Differentiate pseudocysts based on size and symptoms:
  Non-symptomatic pseudocysts less than 4 cm in size should be followed by serial ultrasound/CT scans. You can continue to follow the pseudocysts as long as they are decreasing in size or asymptomatic. Be prepared for the pseudocyst to rupture, obstruct, bleed, get secondarily infected, or increase in size.

Most pseudocysts are now thought to resolve over time. There is no longer a minimum size to drain an asymptomatic pseudocyst. Use serial imaging instead. Once the wall has matured, if the pseudocyst causes symptoms, the patient has frequent bouts of pancreatitis, or there are concerns for malignancy, consider surgical treatment.

1. Perform ERCP to see if it communicates:
   (a) If does not communicate, you can consider CT aspiration (~40 % success rate) or leaving a catheter in the cyst cavity (on the boards, these options will fail and cause pancreaticocutaneous fistula, or the cyst will get secondarily infected).
   (b) If it does communicate and is symptomatic, then perform surgical drainage.
2. Choices for internal drainage (pseudocyst wall takes about 6 weeks to mature):
   (a) Cystgastrostomy: Perform anterior gastrostomy, palpation, and needle aspiration to find the cyst in the back wall of stomach. Then open the cyst, <u>send part of the wall for biopsy</u>, and suture the posterior wall of the stomach to the mature cyst wall. The opening should be 5 cm. Use interrupted absorbable sutures.
   (b) Cystojejunostomy: Use a Roux loop when the cyst is not adherent to the posterior wall of the stomach. You can check this by opening the gastrocolicomentum and seeing if there is a plane between the posterior stomach and cyst or multiple cysts (using side-to-side anastomosis).
   (c) Cystoduodenostomy: If pseudocyst is in the head of the pancreas close to the duodenum, use a Kocher maneuver to check. Make a 3-cm opening into the first or third portion of the duodenum using a transduodenal approach.
   (d) Distal pancreatectomy: This is an option if the pseudocyst is in the pancreatic tail or has eroded into surrounding structures.
3. External drainage only for the following:
   (a) Infected pseudocysts
   (b) An unstable patient with free rupture or bleed
4. Bleeding in a patient with a pseudocyst can be from:

(a) Bleeding into the bowel from erosion into bowel wall
(b) Bleeding from gastric varices (splenectomy is the treatment of choice here because varices form secondary to splenic vein thrombosis)
(c) Bleeding into the cyst (erosion into one of the pancreatic vessels)
(d) Bleeding from a ruptured pseudoaneurysm (usually splenic artery)
(e) Bleeding may occur into the cyst, into the bowel, or free into the peritoneal cavity
Angiogram is helpful here if the patient is stable enough. Otherwise, perform a laparotomy, ligate offending vessels, open the cyst, pack, and return, or go to angiogram as necessary.

Common Curveballs

Patient has multiple cysts
The examiner tries to get you to change your management strategy, so the size may change during the questioning from 4 to 8 cm
The examiner tries to get you to operate before a mature wall has formed
Pseudocyst ruptures into the thoracic cavity (pancreatic hydrothorax—drain effusion, TPN, and stent if needed)
Your first choice of internal drainage is not an option (prior surgery, etc.)
Patient with known pseudocyst develops bleeding into the pseudocyst and presents in shock (see above for differential diagnosis—perform angiogram to embolize bleeding vessel; otherwise, perform an exploratory laparotomy, ligation of splenic or gastroduodenal artery, then open and pack cyst and ligate bleeders within the cyst wall)
The pseudocyst gets infected if you tried to aspirate it
Patient gets a pancreatic fistula if you left a drainage catheter for a noncommunicating cyst
Gastroenterologist is not available for ERCP or endoscopic cystgastrostomy
Endoscopic cystgastrostomy results in free perforation/bleeding at the anastomotic site

Biopsy of the wall reveals malignancy
Patient has a pancreatitis flare after ERCP
Pseudocyst is actually a cystic neoplasm as shown by intraoperative frozen section biopsy (scenario switch!)
Patient who you decided to follow develops a complication from the pseudocyst, such as the following:
Cyst rupture—pancreatic ascites
Infection (fever, increasing WBC, increasing abdominal pain—perform open surgical drainage)
Bleeding (hemorrhagic shock)
Duodenal obstruction
Pseudoaneurysm
Splenic vein thrombosis

Clean Kills

Forgetting to biopsy the wall of the pseudocyst
Not waiting for wall to mature
Not obtaining a CT scan
Not knowing how to perform internal drainage procedure
Not getting a preoperative ERCP to determine if pseudocyst communicates with the pancreatic duct
Taking a patient with bleeding from the pseudocyst to surgery rather than angiogram to embolize offending vessel
Mentioning laparoscopic cystgastrostomy (although it has been performed by several authors, do *not* mention it!)

Summary

Pseudocysts can often occur after bouts of pancreatitis. Remember, differential diagnosis can also include mucinous adenoma, AAA, or other intra-abdominal masses. There is a movement now to treat pseudocysts mainly for symptoms and not necessarily size. Be sure to wait 6 weeks for the wall to mature prior to surgery. ERCP with stenting may be a less invasive treatment option. Send a piece of the wall when performing a cyst-gastrostomy to rule out other diagnoses.

Pediatric

Linda Szczurek

Neonatal Bowel Obstruction

Concept

Bilious vomiting is!) always a surgical emergency in the newborn. Multiple possible etiologies exist, including annular pancreas, duodenal web, malrotation, jejunoileal atresia, meconium ileus, Hirschsprung's disease, infection/necrotizing enterocolitis, and metabolic abnormalities (K+, Mg++).

Always look for associated anomalies such as cystic fibrosis (meconium ileus) and trisomy 21 (duodenal atresia, malrotation).

Way Question May Be Asked?

"You are called to the neonatal intensive care unit (NICU) to evaluate a baby that has had bilious vomiting since birth. What do you want to do?"

Always look for congenital anomalies, Down's stigmata, and remember that this is a surgical emergency.

How to Answer?

History
    Maternal polyhydramnios
    Onset of bilious emesis (with every feeding)
    Delayed meconium passage
    Prematurity
    Family history

Physical Examination
    Evidence of dehydration (sunken fontanelle, skin turgor)
    Abdominal distension or scaphoid abdomen
    Any congenital anomalies (imperforate)
Diagnostic Tests
    "Babygram"—look for pattern of the gas
    "Double bubble"—duodenal atresia or malrotation with volvulus
    Dilated small bowel loops—jejunoileal atresia
    Upper gastrointestinal (UGI) series if you suspect proximal obstruction or malrotation
    Barium enema (BE) if you suspect distal obstruction

Surgical Treatment

1. Administer nothing by mouth, intravenous fluids (IVF), nasogastric tube (NGT) and correct electrolytes.
2. Determine if obstruction is <u>proximal or distal.</u>
3. Go to the operating room (OR) if there is any evidence of peritonitis.
4. For duodenal atresia, proceed to the OR once patient is resuscitated.
   (a) Perform duodenojejunostomy through a transverse right upper quadrant (RUQ) incision.
   (b) Obstruction is usually immediately post-ampullary.
   (c) Insert a gastrostomy tube (G-tube).
5. Malrotation (often associated with diaphragmatic hernia, abdominal wall defects, and jejunoileal atresia)
   (a) Perform counterclockwise detorsion if volvulus is present.
   (b) Take a second look if there is questionable viability.
   (c) Perform Ladd's procedure:
       Divide the peritoneal bands crossing the duodenum (extending from the ligament of Trietz).
       Position the duodenum and jejunum to the right of midline.
       Position the colon to the left of midline.
       Perform an incidental appendectomy.

L. Szczurek, D.O., F.A.C.O.S. (✉)
General Surgery Department, Kennedy Health System,
2201 Chapel Avenue West, Suite 100, Cherry Hill, NJ 08002, USA
e-mail: lszczurek@hotmail.com

M.A. Neff (ed.), *Passing the General Surgery Oral Board Exam,*
DOI 10.1007/978-1-4614-7663-4_10 © Springer Science+Business Media New York 2014

(d) Treat other anomalies if present.

(e) Cecopexy/duodenopexy is not necessary.

6. Jejunoileal atresia (the more distal the obstruction, the more abdominal distension the child will have)

(a) Administer a BE to document normal colon.

(b) Resect the atretic portion.

(c) Inject saline to make sure there is no distal obstruction (web/atresia).

(d) Perform end-to-end anastomosis.

7. Duodenal web

(a) Perform a longitudinal duodenotomy.

(b) Perform a partial membrane excision.

8. Meconium ileus—failure to pass meconium in <24 h with bilious emesis, abdominal distension, and perforated anus (produces obstruction from inspissated meconium secondary to pancreatic exocrine insufficiency)

(a) Evaluate for cystic fibrosis.

(b) Look for ground glass appearance on abdominal x-ray instead of air fluid (A/F) levels.

(c) Administer gastrograffin enema, pancreatic enzymes by NGT, and acetylcysteine (Mucomyst) for an uncomplicated presentation.

(d) For a complicated meconium ileus, proceed to the OR:
Resect the nonviable bowel.
Repair perforations.
Drain any abscesses.
Perform enterotomy plus an injection of acetylcysteine.

Common Curveballs

The "double bubble" seen on x-ray is malrotation and not duodenal obstruction

Scenario switches from proximal to distal obstruction

Patient has multiple atretic areas in jejunum/ileum

Patient has the appearance of total small bowel infarction

Patient has associated anomalies (only cardiac anomalies affect your decision to operate)

Clean Kills

Not identifying malrotation

Not knowing Ladd's bands or details of Ladd's procedure

Not knowing what "double bubble" means on "babygram"

Not looking for associated anomalies

Not treating bilious vomiting as a surgical emergency

Pyloric Stenosis

Concept

Pyloric stenosis is thickening of the muscle of the pylorus resulting in functional outlet obstruction. It is the most common surgical cause of emesis in infants. Etiology is unknown, but it is more common in first-born males.

Way Question May Be Asked?

"You are called to the ED to evaluate a 9-week-old infant with a history of intermittent nonbilious emesis that is now projectile vomiting. What do you want to do?" You may be given an infant with clear signs of dehydration or it may be an older child (up to 2 years old). The key is whether or not the vomiting was bilious.

How to Answer?

History
   Sex (male > female)
   Age (2–8 weeks)
   FHx Family history of pyloric stenosis
   Bilious vs. nonbilious vomiting
   Vomiting of undigested formula shortly after feeding
   Intermittent emesis progressing to projectile
   Infant is hungry between episodes of vomiting
Physical Examination
   Sunken fontanelle
   Dry mucous membranes
   Decreased skin turgor
Abdominal Examination
   Thickened pylorus or "olive" in epigastrum (need infant to be quiet and stomach empty)
   Observation of gastric peristaltic waves
Diagnostic Tests
   Full laboratory panels, especially K + (hypokalemic, hypochloremic metabolic alkalosis)
   Ultrasound (elongated pyloric channel, thickened pyloric diameter, increased pyloric wall thickness)
   Barium UGI (elongated narrow pyloric channel—"string sign", gastric outlet obstruction)

Surgical Treatment

1. Correct electrolyte abnormalities (this is an elective surgical procedure!)
2. D51/2NS + 20 KCl
3. Pyloromyotomy (Ramstedt technique):
   Perform under general anesthesia.
   Place an NGT (especially if UGI) to avoid aspiration.
   Make a transverse epigastric or RUQ incision.
   Grasp the pylorus between two fingers.
   Make an incision with the scalpel into the serosa/muscle.
   Use the back of the scalpel handle to blunt complete pyloromyotomy.
   You should see a bulging mucosa.
   Be careful not to perforate the underlying mucosa. If it perforates, close and cover with an omental patch. Alternatively, close the myotomy, rotate the pylorus 45 degrees, and perform the pyloromyotomy again.
   Check for leak by putting a small amount of air through the NGT.
4. You can start feeding 6–12 h postoperatively with dilute milk and advance as tolerated.
5. Small episodes of emesis are not uncommon in the immediate postoperative period (can be due to gastrointestinal reflux disease, discordant peristalsis, or gastric atony). Pursue with a UGI series to check for an incomplete pyloromyotomy if it extends past postoperative day 2.

Common Curveballs

Patient has low potassium (how will you manage?)

Examiner asks when you will start feeding the child

Patient has mucosal perforation during your pyloromyotomy (now what?)

Patient has malrotation, antral web, or duodenal stenosis (scenario switch)

Pyloromyotomy is incomplete

Examiner asks you to describe paradoxic aciduria (Vomiting leads to loss of fluid with high K+, H+, and Cl⁻ concentrations. Volume deficit leads to aldosterone-mediated Na+ resorption with loss of K+. The body tries to hold onto K+, leading to excretion of H+ ions that leads to paradoxicaciduria, It is treated by replacing volume before administering K+!)

Examiner asks how to calculate the volume of fluid to be administered to the infant, given a weight in kilograms (4 cc/kg/h for the first 10 kg, 2 cc/kh/h for the second 10 kg, and 1 cc/kg/h for every kilogram after)

Clean Kills

Mistaking the diagnosis for one of the many etiologies for neonatal bowel obstruction

Not being able to describe how to resuscitate the patient preoperatively

Describing laparoscopic pyloromyotomy

Not being able to explain the hypokalemic, hypochloremic metabolic alkalosis that typically accompanies these patients

Summary

Pyloric stenosis is due to thickening of the muscle, resulting in a functional outlet obstruction that presents as projectile vomiting. It is most commonly seen in first-born males at age 2–8 weeks. On examination, the infant may have a palpable "olive" in the epigatrum. On laboratory studies, the patient will often have hypokalemic, hypochloremic, metabolic alkalosis. The treatment is correction of the electrolyte abnormalities, IVF, and pyloromyotomy.

Pediatric Inguinal Hernia

Concept

Inguinal hernia repair is the most common operation performed by pediatric surgeons. Hernias are most common in the first year of life and are more common in premature infants, in males, and on the right side. These indirect hernias are due to failure of the processus vaginalis to close during development.

Way Question May Be Asked?

"You are asked to evaluate a 3-month-old male during surgical clinic. His young mother is very nervous. The other day while she was bathing him, the infant began crying and she noticed a lump in his right groin. He was born a few weeks premature but is otherwise in good health. What do you want to do?"

The key is getting a very good history from the mother and trying to reproduce the bulge on examination.

How to Answer?

History
  Prematurity
  Sex (more common in males than females)
  Side of lump (more common on right than left)
  Timing (is the lump present all the time or does it stick out when the baby increases abdominal pressure?)
Physical Examination
  Examine for inguinal mass or asymmetry
  Palpate cord for thickness (silk glove sign)
Diagnostic Tests
  Ultrasound if the examination is inconclusive

Surgical Treatment

Perform open inguinal hernia repair with high ligation of the hernia sac with an absorbable suture.

Common Curveballs

Patient has bilateral hernias (always check for this)
Patient has injury to the vas deferens (can be repaired with 8-0 monofilament absorbable suture at the time of injury

Clean Kills

Waiting to repair the hernia (this can lead to incarceration or strangulation)
Not identifying the hernia
Attempting to put mesh in an infant/child or not knowing the proper technique for repair in a child
Confusing a hydrocele for a hernia

Tracheoesophageal fistula

Concept

Tracheoesophageal fistula (TEF) is a common cause of respiratory distress in infants. Several variants exist:
A. Esophageal atresia and distal TEF (most common)
B. Atresia without fistula
C. H-type TEF
D. Atresia with proximal and distal TEF
  Approximately 50 % of infants will have other congenital defects (VACTERL—vertebral, anorectal, cardiovascular, TEF, renal, limb) and you need to rule these in/out prior to operation.

Way Question May Be Asked?

"You are called to the NICU to evaluate a newborn who is small for his gestational age. He had an episode of choking and desaturation with his first two feedings. What do you want to do?" You should consider TEF in any newborn with respiratory distress. Key to this condition is that the problems are associated with feeding. Most TEFs should be identified pre-term by ultrasound.

How to Answer?

History
  Earliest clinical sign is excessive salivation
  Maternal polyhydramnios
  Respiratory distress with first feeding (choking, coughing, regurgitation)
  Desaturation with nippling
Physical Examination
  Cannot place NGT
  Small for gestational age
  Scaphoid abdomen (if atresia without TEF)
  Imperforated anus or limb abnormalities
  Cardiac examination
Diagnostic Tests
  "Babygram"(air in the GI tract rules out atresia without TEF; rule out duodenal atresia, vertebral anomalies)
  0.5 cc barium down NGT (blunt pouch)
  Preoperative echocardiogram to rule out cardiac anomalies (affects anesthesia management)
  Renal ultrasound before or after repair
  Chromosomal analysis

Surgical Treatment

1. Place NGT in pouch (to prevent aspiration pneumonitis).
2. Elevate head of bed (to prevent aspiration pneumonitis).
3. Adminster antibiotics if pneumonia.
4. Administer IVF.
5. Proceed to the OR in the first 24–48 h for repair:
   (a) Use an extrapleural approach through a right thoracotomy.
   (b) Divide the fistula.
   (c) Close the trachea.
   (d) Perform end-to-end esophageal anastomosis.
   (e) Use gastrotomy for early postoperative feeding.
   (f) Leave a drain next to the esophageal anastomosis.
   (g) An alternative is gastrotomy only: Create a spit fistula in the neck and delay repair until the patient is 1 year old (colon interposition is usually performed in cases of atresia without TEF).

Common Curveballs

Patient has postoperative complications:

Leak (13–16 %: if a drain is left, 95 % will close spontaneously; you can also use a pleural or pericardial patch with or without an intercostal muscle flap)

Stricture (up to 80 %: use balloon dilatation; if it fails, patient may require resection and reanastamosis)

Recurrent fistula (3–14 %: due to leak and inflammation and erosion through previous repair site; can also use a flap)

Reflux (30–70 %: treat medically)

You enter the pleura during an extrapleural approach

Patient has associated anomalies (Down syndrome, valvular defect, etc.)

You are not able to perform primary end-to-end anastomosis because of a long "gap"

Patient presents with an H-type fistula (repeated episodes of pneumonia in infancy)

Patient has an associated imperforate anus (scenario switch)

Clean Kills

Not making the diagnosis

Not knowing the most common type/how to repair most common type

Not ruling other associated anomalies preoperatively (especially cardiac!)

Not trying to place NGT (alternatively, continuing to try to advance when meet resistance)

Not placing G-tube at operation

Summary

Tracheoesophageal fistulas come in several variants, the most common being esophageal atresia with a distal TEF. Approximately 50 % of infants with a TEF have other associated congenital defects that must be ruled out prior to surgery. The most common presenting symptoms are excessive salivation and respiratory distress with the first feeding. An NGT is unable to be placed on physical examination. X-ray can help narrow down the type of atresia/TEF. The exact surgical technique depends on the type of fistula, but a G-tube for early feeding should be placed. The overall survival rate is 85–95 %.

Perioperative Care

Jonathan Nguyen and Marc A. Neff

Hypotension in the Recovery Room

Concept

With hypotension in the recovery room, it is easy to get lost in the myriad of possible diagnoses. The key is being methodical and stepwise. Approach the patient like a trauma patient, working through your ABCs. Differential diagnosis (DDx) includes any form of shock—hypovolemic shock (inadequate fluids intraoperatively), hemorrhagic shock (patient is still bleeding), cardiogenic shock (myocardial infarction [MI], pneumothorax)—as well as sepsis (unlikely so quick), transfusion reaction, malignant hyperthermia, Addisonian crisis, and air/fat embolism.

Way Question May Be Asked?

"You are called to evaluate a 63-year-old man after an abdominal aortic aneurysm (AAA) repair. He was stable in the recovery room for about 2 h and now his blood pressure (BP) has dropped to 80/40. What do you want to do?"

The question could be asked in many different ways, with the patient's status post any major abdominal operation. The patient may have received blood intraoperatively. You may or may not be given other vital signs at the start.

J. Nguyen, D.O. (✉)
General Surgery, University of Medicine & Dentistry of New Jersey, Stratford, NJ, USA
e-mail: diligenceb@yahoo.com

M.A. Neff, M.D., F.A.C.S.
Minimally Invasive, 2201 Chapel Avenue West, Suite 100, Cherry Hill, NJ 08002, USA
e-mail: mneffyhs@aol.com

How to Answer?

Be methodical! Work through your ABCs while resuscitating the patient:

Airway
  Is the patient on a ventilator?
  What is the respiratory rate and pulse oximetry?
  Does the patient need to be intubated?

Breathing
  Are both lung sounds present?
  Does the patient need a chest tube?

Circulation
  Check pulses.
  Are extremities cold (hypovolemic shock) or warm (anaphylactic)?

Ample History
  Type of procedure
  Length of surgery
  Fluids/blood
  Previous/past medical history
  Was a central venous pressure (CVP) line placed intraoperatively?

Physical Examination
  Vital signs (fever is very suggestive)
  Neck veins (flat or distended)
  Heart rate (arrythmia)
  Rash (petechiae with transfusion reaction)
  Generalized oozing (disseminated intravascular coagulation)
  Pulses in extremities
  Abdominal examination

Surgical Treatment

1. Order

   Chest x-ray (CXR), electrocardiogram (EKG), arterial blood gas (ABG), complete laboratory panel, and urinalysis.

   Send the patient's blood along with transfused bags if you suspect a transfusion reaction (also check urine for hemoglobin [Hgb]).

2. CVP or Swanz Ganz Catheter (SGC) to direct fluid management

3. Treat specific underlying problem

   (a) For hypovolemic shock: fluid resuscitation

   (b) For cardiogenic shock: SGC plus pressors

   (c) For pneumothorax: chest tube

   (d) For malignant hyperthermia: cooling, supportive care, and <u>dantrolene</u>

   (e) For Addisonian crisis: bolus steroids (100 mg hydrocortisone)

   (f) For air/fat embolism: supportive care

   (g) For transfusion reaction: key is to keep up Urine output (UO) and avoid precipitation of Hgb in renal tubules

   Fluids to maintain UO: 100 cc/h

   2 amps bicarbonate plus add to IVF to alkalinize urine (check pH > 7)

   Mannitol (1–2 mg/kg) (osmotic diuretic)

Common Curveballs

Patient has MI and you are asked about your management/pressors

Patient has refractory hypotension to anything you do

Patient has a transfusion reaction and you are asked your specific management, including how to alkalinize the urine

Patient needs to be intubated

Patient needs CVP/SGC

You are given a set of SGC parameters to interpret

Patient develops renal failure (change scenario)

Clean Kills

Taking patient back to the OR (usually, they are not trying to get you o take the patient back to the OR)

Not being methodical and going through ABCs:

   Missed mucus plug

   Missed pneumothorax from a CVP line that the anesthesiologist placed

   Missed kinked endotracheal tube

Missing vital signs (fever and hypotension point you in some specific directions)

Postoperative Fever

Concept

Postoperative fever has multiple causes, so you should be systematic. Remember the number of postoperative days and the most common causes. Never forget to check the wound for a necrotizing soft tissue infection or change the CVP for possible line sepsis. Differential diagnosis includes the following:

<u>Days 0–2</u>: atelectasis, necrotizing soft tissue infection

<u>Days 3–5</u>: Urinary tract infection, pneumonia

<u>Days 5–7</u>: Wound infection/abscess

<u>Days 7–10</u>: Deep vein thrombosis (DVT), anastomotic leak, *Clostridium difficile*

Immediate postoperative period: Addisonian crisis, thyrotoxicosis

Anytime: line sepsis, drug fever, transfusion reaction (soon after transfusion: red blood cells, platelets, fresh frozen plasma, cryoprecipitate)

Way Question May Be Asked?

"You are called to see a patient 3 days after a right hemicolectomy for an adenomatous polyp. The patient is febrile to 101.4. What do you want to do?"

The scenario may be after any operation and any number of days postoperatively. The key is to resuscitate the unstable patient in the intensive care unit (ICU), perform a complete examination with attention to the wound and intravenous (IV) sites, get appropriate diagnostic tests, and then be aggressive with the management when appropriate. Common scenarios will include necrotizing soft tissue infection, anastomotic leak, enterocutaneous fistula, and intraabdominal abscess.

How to Answer?

History

   Type of surgery (how dirty was the case?)

   Antibiotic use

   Recent transfusions

   Associated symptoms (cough, chills, rigors, pain, dysuria, diarrhea)

   IV sites (how old)

   Immunosuppression (transplantation, human immunodeficiency virus, chemotherapy, steroid use?)

Physical

   Vital signs (shock?)

   Complete physical examination

Wound
IV sites
Foley catheter?

Diagnostic Tests
Complete laboratory panels (including complete blood count with differential, liver function tests, amylase, urinalysis)
Culture and Gram stain for any wound drainage
Low threshold to open up any wounds
Sputum Gram stain/culture
Blood cultures (useful only if your patient is still alive 48 h later when the results return!)
CXR
± CT scan (to rule out abscess)
± Duplex ultrasound of lower extremities
± Thyroid hormone levels
± Stool for *C. difficile* toxin assay

Surgical Treatment

1. Low threshold to open wound
2. Low threshold to change CVP and send tip for culture
3. Low threshold to transfer unstable patient to ICU
4. For a necrotizing wound infection:
   (a) Open the wound.
   (b) Obtain a Gram stain and Culture and sensitivity (C+S).
   (c) Take the patient immediately to the operating room (OR).
   (d) Perform a wide debridement to viable tissue.
   (e) Close with a vacuum-assisted closure sponge, Bogata bag, cadaveric skin, or pack.
   (f) Return to OR the following day to repeat debridement, and then daily until only viable tissue remains.
   (g) Treat with penicillin G or broad-spectrum antibiotics based on Gram stain and cultures
   (h) Typical organisms include Clostridia, Streptococcus, and mixed infections.
5. For a retained foreign body:
   (a) Obtain an abdominal x-ray/CXR ± CT scan to identify the foreign body.
   (b) Promptly take the patient to the OR.
   (c) Examiner may ask how you will describe the situation to the patient and family. (Honesty is the best policy!)

Common Curveballs

Patient has a necrotizing wound infection (how will you manage?)
Patient has a retained foreign body left behind from surgery

Examiner asks how you will discuss a retained foreign body with the patient and family
Examiner asks how to treat/close the wound for a patient with a necrotizing infection
Patient has *C. difficile* enterocolitis and needs emergent abdominal surgery
Examiner asks about your antibiotic selection and why
Scenario switches on you from postoperative day (POD) 2 to POD 5 to POD 10
Patient has an anastomotic leak
Patient has a fistula
Patient has an intra-abdominal abscess
Patient has a transfusion reaction
Patient has an Addisonian Crisis
Patient has thyrotoxicosis
Patient has a DVT

Clean Kills

Getting lost in discussions about paraneoplastic syndromes, subacute bacterial endocarditis, drug fever, parotitis, or otitis
Pursuing a workup for sinusitis and acalculous cholecystitis in any patient other than a debilitated patient in the ICU
Not considering line sepsis
Not evaluating the wound
Not recognizing and appropriately treating a necrotizing wound infection
Waiting for blood culture results before making any definitive management decisions

Postoperative Myocardial Infarction

Concept

With the increasing age and comorbidities of the population, MIs are becoming increasingly more common. Because patients are usually anesthetized for surgery, silent MI may occur more frequently than previously believed or it may be masked by postoperative pain. Risk factors are age >75 years, acute decompensated heart failure, coronary artery disease (CAD), and planned vascular procedure.

Way Question May Be Asked?

"An 87-year-old male smoker with CAD underwent an exploratory laparotomy for feculent diverticulitis. During recovery, he is in pain and his pulse is 96 bpm. ST depressions are noted on his EKG." How do you proceed?

How to Answer?

Perioperative myocardial infarction (PMI) mortality ranges from 10 % to 15 %, similar to non-PMI mortality. There are five types of MI: traditional MI, MI secondary to increased demand or decreased supply, cardiac death, MI after percutaneous coronary intervention (PCI), and MI after coronary artery bypass grafting (CABG).

PMIs are usually caused by a combination of induced stress (catecholamine surge, pain, increased demand) and unstable plaques being broken off. This can occur anywhere from intraoperatively to postoperative day 3. PMIs are usually silent, masked by anesthesia and pain. Mild elevations in heart rate and >10 min of intermittent ST depression may be the only indicators.

1. Work through the ABCs: Check the patient's vital signs and assess hemodynamic stability.
2. Does patient have any symptoms of chest pain, arm pain, jaw pain, blurred vision, etc.?
3. Check EKG and serial cardiac enzymes (CEs) over the next 6–9 h.
4. Creatine kinase MB is elevated in first few hours postoperatively (quicker release) and cardiac troponins are elevated over hours to days (delayed release).
5. Consult a cardiologist if the EKG/CEs are indicative of an MI.
6. If an ST segment elevation myocardial infarction (STEMI) or unstable non-ST segment elevation myocardial infarction (NSTEMI) is identified, proceed to PCI knowing that if treatment is rendered, the patient will require acetylsalicylic acid (ASA, 325 mg) ± clopidogrel (Plavix) and heparin drip.
7. If the patient is unstable, transfuse to a hemoglobin level >10 and administer dobutamine if needed.
8. For a stable NSTEMI, treat conservatively. Start ASA (325 mg). If risk of surgical site bleeding is acceptable, start a heparin drip. Enoxaparin (Lovenox) has a higher risk of bleeding (longer half-life) and must be renal dosed in kidney disease. Control pain. If the patient's BP/heart rate can tolerate it, start beta-blocker (decreased demand), statin (plaque stabilization), and angiotensin-converting-enzyme inhibitor (ACE-I, prevents remodeling).

Remember the stable NSTEMI pneumonic: MONA-BASH (morphine, oxygen, nitroglycerin, ASA, beta-blocker, ACE-I, statin, heparin drip).

Common Curveballs

The examiner asks which anticoagulant should be started (heparin drip is easier to reverse and does not require renal dosing)

Knowing what to administer for a right-sided MI (do not give morphine or nitroglycerin)

Clean Kills

Not checking EKG
Not checking CEs
Not considering a pulmonary embolism
Not considering ASA or heparin drip

Summary

Perioperative MIs are becoming more frequent as patients are living longer with more complicated medical comorbidities. Early diagnosis is usually achieved by high clinical suspicion (tachycardia and ST depressions) and confirmed with EKG/CE changes. Assess the patient's stability. If STEMI or unstable, proceed to PCI. If the patient is stable, medically manage with MONA-BASH.

Recent Myocardial Infarction

Concept

Many patients will have elevated operative risk given cardiac history. Risk factors include hypertension, diabetes mellitus, angina, vascular disease, and family history.

Way Question May Be Asked?

"A 56-year-old male is a heavy smoker who had a recent MI. He now presents with signs and symptoms consistent with acute cholecystitis."

The question may concern any common general surgery issue, with the patient having had a recent MI.

The examiners may actually throw the scenario at you where the patient has multiple problems, such as obstructing or bleeding rectal cancer, as well as having had a recent MI.

How to Answer?

Know the important Goldman criteria: aortic stenosis, MI within 6 months, emergency surgery, nonsinus rhythm, age >70 years, jugular venous distension, poor medical condition (PO$_2$ <60, CR >3.0, chronic liver disease); class 3 has a 14 % risk and Class 4 has a 78 % risk.

Emergency operations performed without cardiac preparation have an up to 5 % perioperative risk of MI.

No type of anesthesia (local, epidural, or general) is better than any other when administered by a good anesthesiologist.

Obtain a preoperative workup as best as possible to determine cardiac status (EKG, CXR, echocardiogram for ejection fraction)

An asymptomatic patient who received CABG/PCI <5 years ago and with noninvasive study <2 years ago is low risk for surgery.

If find a reversible defect on stress thallium, perform a cardiac catheterization.

If you find a lesion, have a bypass/PCI performed.

If the patient is on beta-blockers for >1 month, continue them throughout hospitalization. Do not start perioperatively unless the patient has suffered an MI.

Stop ASA/Plavix 5–7 days prior to surgery.

Use preoperative SGC, nitroglycerin drip, and maximize hemodynamics.

Invasive Monitoring

A patient with conduction system disease may require temporary pacemaker support during surgery.

Bare metal stent (risk of 10 % if <30 days and 2.8 % if >90 days)

Drug-eluding stents (risk ~6 % for the first year and 3.3 % for >1 year)

Perioperative mortality is ~10 % with the following:

(a) Recent MI (risk ~30 % if less than 30 days, 6 % if less than 3 months, 2 % if 3–6 months)
(b) Acute decompensated heart failure
(c) Unstable angina
(d) Severe valvular disease (less than 0.9 cm^2 for aortic valve and 1.5 cm^2 for mitral valve)

Common Curveballs

Patient has a perioperative MI (see section on Postoperative Myocardial Infarction)

Patient has perioperative arrhythmias (atrial fibrillation is particularly popular as a complication in any scenario whether recent MI or not—do not forget your Advanced Cardiovascular Life Support!)

Patient has postoperative pulmonary edema (usually from perioperative fluid shifts; may need pulmonary capillary wedge pressure [PCWP] to assess volume status)

Examiner asks how you will manage the patient preoperatively

Clean Kills

Not knowing any of the Goldman criteria

Not adequately working up patient preoperatively

Forgetting about intraoperative monitoring

Believing that one type of anesthesia superior to another—the risk itself is just anesthesia, so do the surgery you need to do

Not appropriately dealing with postoperative complications

Summary

Surgery in patients with high cardiac risk is becoming more common. Conduct a preoperative evaluation with EKG, two-dimensional echocardiogram, and stress test if needed. Perform PCWP if further information on heart function is required. Remember Goldman's criteria for risk stratification.

Renal Failure

Concept

Renal failure has multiple causes, but it can be broken down into pre-renal, intra-renal, and post-renal causes. Certain information on the history and physical examination, along with your diagnostic tests, will help you here.

Differential Diagnosis

Pre-renal

Hypovolemic shock

Hemorrhagic shock

Septic shock

Third space losses (burns, pancreatitis, long operation, cirrhosis)

Vascular (emboli, renal artery occlusion)

Abdominal compartment syndrome

Intra-renal

Acute tubular necrosis—from ischemia, secondary to inadequate perfusion (from pre-renal cause above)

Acute interstitial nephritis—secondary to medication (penicillin)

Post-renal

Urethral obstruction (catheter/prostate)

Bilateral ureteral obstruction (intraoperative injury, retroperitoneal fibrosis)

You always want to convert oliguric renal failure into nonoliguric renal failure. Most often, the cause will be hypovolemia in surgical patients.

Way Question May Be Asked?

"You are called to see a patient 6 h after AAA repair. The patient's urine output has been 15 cc the past 3 h. What do you want to do?"

The question may occur after any operation or in the management of any patient, such as after multiple trauma, burns, or abdominoperineal resection.

How to Answer?

History
  Intake/output
  Intraoperative fluids
  Clamp time on AAA (suprarenal or infrarenal)
  History of renal disease
  Nephrotoxic meds
  Diuretic use
  Recent transfusions (hemolysis with precipitation in renal tubules)
  Trauma with major muscle injury (myoglobinuria)

Physical
  Vital signs (shock?)
  Skin (turgor?)
  Mucous membranes
  Chest (congestive heart failure [CHF]?)
  Abdomen (distended bladder?)
  Check Foley catheter (is one in place? has it been flushed?)
  Bladder pressures (for abdominal compartment syndrome)

Diagnostic Tests
  Complete laboratory panels
  Blood urea nitrogen/creatinine ratio
  Urinalysis (protein with glomerular disease, eosinophils with interstitial nephritis)
  Urinary electrolytes (urinary sodium < 20 suggests prerenal etiology)
  Ultrasound to evaluate kidneys
    Obstruction
    Confirm two kidneys
  CVP or SGC to determine volume status
  ± Intravenous pyelogram to evaluate kidney function confirm no post-renal obstruction(be carefulof die load, use non-nephrotoxic contrast agents)
  ± Renal scan—MAG3 scan, useful to assess kidney perfusion

Surgical Treatment

1. Maintain a <u>low threshold</u> for CVP, <u>transfer to ICU</u>, and SGC.
2. Discontinue any nephrotoxic drugs and supplemental potassium.
3. Go through your DDx for renal failure.
4. Perform fluid resuscitation and monitor hourly urine output.
5. Administer dopamine at renal doses.
6. Administer furosemide (Lasix) to convert to nonoliguric renal failure.
7. ± Administer mannitol.
8. Monitor electrolytes closely.
9. Consider dialysis.

Common Curveballs

Examiner asks you about the indications for dialysis.
Examiner asks you to describe how to measure bladder pressures and their significance
Examiner asks you how to treat abdominal compartment syndrome
Patient is unresponsive to all resuscitative measures
Patient has myoglobinuria (how will you manage? alkalinize urine)
Patient has a transfusion reaction and develops renal failure (how will you manage?)
Patient has only one kidney
Patient does not respond to fluid boluses
Patient is elderly with brittle heart, is prone to CHF, or has a low ejection fraction
You are unable to place a Foley catheter
Patient has hematuria

Clean Kills

Not breaking DDx down into pre-renal, intra-renal, and post-renal causes
Not placing at least CVP after two fluid boluses without a response
Not being aggressive with resuscitation of the patient
Not identifying abdominal compartment syndrome
Performing an angiogram acutely
Performing a renal biopsy acutely

Skin and Soft Tissue

Marc A. Neff

Melanoma

Concept

There are four main subtypes of melanoma—superficial spreading, nodular, lentigomaligna, and acrallentigenous—with several special situations (anal, subungal). Your workup must be systematic—establish risk factors, biopsy, stage the patient, sample lymph nodes, and then determine any adjuvant treatment. Expect questions regarding lymph node sampling, especially groin dissections.

Way Question May Be Asked?

"A 52-year-old man presents to your office with the complaint of a skin lesion on his leg that has recently changed in both color and size."

The question may concern any part of the body. You may also be shown a picture of an obvious melanoma. The patient may have been sent to you after a biopsy performed by a dermatologist.

How to Answer?

Always take a history first:
  Changing skin lesion (A-asymmetry, B-border irregularity, C-color, D-diameter, E-elevation mnemonic)
  Bleeding lesion
  Ulceration
  Itching

Also, establish risk factors for melanoma:
  Excessive sun exposure
  Fair skin
  Positive family history
  History of melanoma
  Dysplastic nevus syndrome
  Xeroderma pigmentosum

Complete Physical Examination
  Examination of lesion (color, size, symmetry)
  Examination of regional lymph node basins

Consider the differential diagnosis:
  Benign nevus
  Seborrheic keratosis
  Pigmented wart
  Squamous cell cancer
  Basal cell cancer

Biopsy
If it is not in a cosmetically sensitive place, excise with a 1- to 2-mm margin.
If it is large, perform a punch biopsy through the thickest portion of the lesion or an incisional biopsy.
Always orient the specimen.
If it is subungal, split open the nail (only need diagnosis here).
  Staging Clark's system has really fallen out of favor. Staging is now mostly based on Breslow depth.

TNM system:
  I: Primary <1.5 mm depth, no nodes
  II: >1.5 mm depth, no nodes
  III: Regional nodal disease or in-transit metastases
  IV: Distant metastases

Histological Staging (Breslow)
Thin: 0–75 mm
Intermediate: 0.76–4 mm
Thick: >4 mm (80 % chance of metastases)

M.A. Neff, M.D., F.A.C.S. (✉)
Minimally Invasive and Bariatric Surgeon,
2201 Chapel Avenue West, Suite 100, Cherry Hill, NJ 08002, USA
e-mail: mneffyhs@aol.com

M.A. Neff (ed.), *Passing the General Surgery Oral Board Exam*,
DOI 10.1007/978-1-4614-7663-4_12, © Springer Science+Business Media New York 2014

Diagnostic Studies

Chest x-ray (CXR)

Laboratory panels—complete blood count, liver function tests, lactate dehydrogenase

Fine needle aspiration (FNA) of any palpable nodes

If there are palpable nodes, perform a computed tomography (CT) scan to evaluate the nodal and next nodal basin, liver, and brain

Margins of Resection You will likely need to re-excise after biopsy.
    5 mm for in-situ lesions
    1 cm for <1 mm depth
    2 cm for >1 mm depth

Head/neck—twice the diameter of the lesion

Subungal finger—split nail to biopsy, amputate distal phalanx (elective node dissection if >0.75 mm)

Subungal toe—ray amputation

Ear—full-thickness wedge resection twice the diameter of the lesion

Anal—local excision, abdominoperineal resection only if the patient is incontinent or has severe pain from invasion of the sphincters

Anterior to ear—re-excision plus modified radical neck dissection and superficial parotidectomy

Lymph Node Sampling

Sentinel lymph node (SLN) biopsy should be offered to all patients with extremity and truncal primaries greater than 1 mm in depth (except subungal).

Obtain a preoperative lymphoscintigraphy.

Use a combination of a handheld gamma counter and Lymphazurin blue dye.

Send the sentinel node for frozen section.

Perform a complete node dissection if the sentinel node is positive.

Only perform a deep node dissection in the groin if there is gross disease in the apical nodes (sapheno-femoral/Cloquet's node) or CT shows suspicious iliac adenopathy.
    Do not perform if there is only microscopic disease in the superficial nodes or the CT suggests nodes that are positive to level of aortic bifurcation; it is unlikely to have any therapeutic benefit and can cause severe leg edema.

Perform a prophylactic node dissection if:
    Lesion is 1–4 mm and overlies the primary nodal basin (parotid, inguinal, axillary)
    Lesion >1 mm in head or neck

Adjuvant Therapy
    Patients with stage II melanomas deeper than 4 mm or stage III disease should be offered vaccine or high-dose interferon.

Treatment of In-Transit/Recurrent Disease
    Re-excision, local radiation, and isolated hyperthermic limb perfusion with melphalan and tumor necrosis factor (TNF) has received a lot of attention recently.

Treatment of Stage IV Disease
    Isolated metastases (liver, lung, brain) should be resected assuming there is no other evidence of disease.

Common Curveballs

Melanoma is not on the extremity but rather is on the trunk and preoplymphoscintigraphy lights up several nodal basins

Lymph nodes in the groin are clinically palpable

Sentinel node biopsy does not work

Other melanomas will be present if you do not perform a complete skin survey

Pulmonary/brain metastases occur during the first several years of follow-up of your patient

Depth of lesion is 0.74 or 0.77 mm

Pathology indicates squamous cell or basal cell carcinoma

Patient has in-transit disease

Patient has two melanomas

Patient has microscopic disease in Cloquet's node (will you do deep inguinal dissection?)

Examiner asks how you will manage of subungal/anal melanoma

Patient has a decline in pulse oximetry reading during the operative procedure (typical artificial side effect of blue dye)

Clean Kills

Not being able to justify your reasoning on doing or not doing a deep inguinal node dissection

Performing a shave biopsy or FNA of a suspected melanoma

Not performing a physical examination of the lymph node basins

Not knowing the difference between Clark's levels and Breslow depth

Not knowing the re-excision margins for different depths of melanomas

Not orienting the specimen for the pathologist

Not getting CT to evaluate the next echelon of nodes with palpable nodes clinically

Not performing a SLN biopsy in head and neck, subungal, and anal melanomas

Trying to perform an SLN biopsy when the lesion overlies a lymph node basin

Trying to offer chemotherapy to patients with isolated metastases

Discussing vaccine therapy (experimental)

Sarcoma

Concept

For sarcomas, pathologic type is not as important as size, grade, location, and resection margins. Lymph node involvement is rare. Therefore, lymph node dissections are only done if grossly involved. Chemotherapy is controversial and marginally beneficial.

Way Question May Be Asked?

"A 39-year-old man presents to the office with a growing mass on his right anterior thigh. On examination, it is hard and fixed to the underlying tissues. What do you do?"

The mass may be found in the extremity of a woman after axillary dissection (Stewart-Treeves syndrome) or in a patient with history of radiation.

How to Answer?

Brief History
  Trauma
  Radiation
  Café au lait spots (von Recklinghausen)
  History of prior lymphadenectomy

Physical Examination
  Examination of tumor
  Lymph nodes
  Neurovascular deficit in the affected extremity

Diagnostic Tests
  CXR + magnetic resonance imaging (MRI)/CT for extremity sarcomas; MRI is more helpful in the retroperitoneum to allow evaluation of the inferior vena cava (IVC)

Biopsy Lesion
  If the lesion is less than 3 cm, you may excise it, but do not shell out due to tumor pseudoencapsulation. Aim for a 2-cm margin.
  If the lesion is larger than 3 cm, perform an incisional biopsy parallel to the muscle group (so as not to compromise future resection).
  A core needle biopsy is acceptable, but tattoo the site of biopsy for later excision.
  Ask the pathologist for the histologic grade.

Treatment
  Perform surgical excision for a grossly clear margin.

In an extremity:
  Take a 2-cm margin. Remove an entire muscle group only if necessary.
  Mark the excision site for adjuvant radiotherapy (XRT), which may reduce the incidence of local recurrence.
  You can leave microscopic disease if it preserves vital neurovascular structures. Postoperative XRT will clean up residual disease.
  Extremity arteries are expendable and can be replaced with a vein or conduit.
  The femoral nerve can be sacrificed, but not the sciatic nerve. Generally, you can sacrifice sensory nerves, but try to preserve motor nerves.
  Removing large central extremity veins leaves the patient with severe edema.
  Perform amputative procedures only for joint involvement (hip, knee, elbow, shoulder, pelvis).
  For small-cell sarcomas (Ewing's), you can consider neoadjuvant chemotherapy/XRT to cytoreduce tumors to allow for limb salvage or salvage of vital neurovascular structures (sciatic nerve).
In the retroperitoneum:
  Perform a wide local resection for grossly clear margins only.
  Perform en bloc resection only for organs where sarcoma is clearly invaded.
  Dissect the sarcoma free if it is adherent to an intraabdominal structure.
  There is no indication for use of adjuvant XRT in retroperitoneal sarcomas (too much visceral toxicity).
  Only perform a percutaneous biopsy if there is extensive periaortic adenopathy and the diagnosis is most likely lymphoma.
  You can excise the IVC if it is involved and replace with Gortex if the patient has not already developed sufficient collateral around it.
Pulmonary Metastases
  It is acceptable to remove pulmonary metastases if the primary disease site is controlled and the number of pulmonary metastases is < 8.

Common Curveballs

Retroperitoneal sarcoma abuts or invades multiple intraabdominal organs
Extremity sarcoma invades neurovascular bundle
Patient has local recurrence (re-excise in the extremity if possible or amputate)
Patient develops lung metastases
IVC is invaded in retroperitoneal sarcoma
Patient has an upper extremity sarcoma

Clean Kills

Attempting an FNA of the mass

Performing an incisional biopsy transverse to an underlying muscle group

Trying to treat only with chemotherapy (only small cell sarcomas!)

Removing adjacent organs in the retroperitoneal sarcoma if there is no invasion

Removing an entire muscle group when a clear margin can be achieved with less aggressive surgery

Not attempting a pulmonary metastectomy when a sarcoma recurs

Resecting the sciatic nerve

Not preparing the patient preoperatively for a possible paralyzed leg or amputation in an attempt to perform an adequate resection

Skin Cancer (Other Than Melanoma)

Concept

Usually, this question will be about squamous cell cancer or basal cell cancer. You can consider other types of benign skin lesions in your differential, but the question will be about how to manage the malignant type. Basal cell carcinoma is most common and may present as a nodular, superficial, or ulcerating lesion.

Way Question May Be Asked?

"A 79-year-old farmer presents to the office with a large mass hidden under his baseball cap. On examination, it is raised, friable, and firm, but it does not appear to be fixed to the underlying bone. What do you do?"

The mass may be on the back, arm, face, or other sun-exposed areas.

How to Answer?

Brief History
  Risk factors
    (Excessive) sun exposure
    Radiation
    Inherited skin disorders

  Physical Examination
    Characteristics of lesion (size, shape, color)
    Full skin survey (include axillae, groin, scalp)

Examine lymph node basins related to lesion

Treatment

Briefly consider differential diagnoses and then proceed to surgical excision and a review of pathology.
  Squamous Cell Carcinoma
    Take 5-mm margins for lesions < 2 cm in size
    Take 1-cm margins for lesions > 2 cm in size
    Perform node dissection if there are palpable nodes or Marjolin's ulcer
  Basal Cell Carcinoma
    Take 2-mm margins
  For lesions on the head/neck, you want to resect and close defect with:
    1. Free full-thickness skin graft from behind the ear or base of the neck
    2. Rotation flap
Indications for Mohs Surgery:
  Recurrent basal/squamous cell carcinomas
    Tumors of the face that are invasive into the nasal, periorbital, or periauricular spaces

Adjuvant Treatment (XRT):
  Close margins of resection (<1 mm)
  Neuro/vascular invasion
  Basal/squamous cell carcinoma in the medial canthus of eye/nose
  Lymph node dissection is only performed for
    clinically involved nodes (modified radical neck dissection plus superior parotidectomy if the tumor is invading the parotid)

Common Curveballs

Pathology comes back as melanoma (scenario switch)

Lymph nodes are palpable

Excised lesion recurs

Lesion is on the face and needs a full-thickness skin graft

Tumor is large and ulcerating

Patient has palpable nodes

Tumor is pre-auricular invading parotid gland

Patient has lesion (cancer) that develops in a chronic wound (Marjolin's ulcer)

Clean Kills

Discussing electrodessication and curettage

Discussing Mohs surgery when not indicated

Discussing simply treating with radiation/chemotherapy

Talking about SLN biopsies or elective lymph node dissection

Marc A. Neff and Devin C. Flaherty

Duodenal Ulcer

Concept

The majority of questions will be related to obstruction, bleeding, or perforation. Most ulcers are related to *Helicobacter pylori* or nonsteroidal anti-inflammatory drug (NSAID) use. Nonoperative therapy may be appropriate for initial discovery of an ulcer and for initial bleeding from the ulcer. Be sure to rule out Zollinger-Ellison (ZE) syndrome, ulcerogenic medications, hyperparathyroidism, and antral G-cell hyperplasia when appropriate.

Way Question May Be Asked?

"A 43-year-old man presents to the emergency department (ED) with acute onset of severe epigastric pain with a rigid abdomen on physical examination. Upright abdominal x-ray (AXR) reveals free air."

You are unlikely to get a presentation this classic. Be sure to go through your differential diagnosis (DDx) for epigastric pain, ruling out myocardial infarction (MI) and pancreatitis, or your DDx for upper gastrointestinal (UGI) bleeding if appropriate.

M.A. Neff, M.D., F.A.C.S.
Minimally Invasive, 2201 Chapel Avenue West, Suite 100, Cherry Hill, NJ 08002, USA
e-mail: mneffyhs@aol.com

D.C. Flaherty, D.O., Ph.D. (✉)
General Surgery, University of Medicine and Dentistry of New Jersey, School of Osteopathic Medicine, Stratford, NJ, USA
e-mail: flaherde@umdnj.edu

How to Answer?

History
    NSAID, smoking, ethanol use
    History of ulcer symptoms (chronic history affects your choice of operation!)
    H. pylori treatment
    Family history (MEN I)
    H2 blocker therapy
    Foreign body ingestion
    Diarrhea (gastrinoma)

History should also focus on symptoms, being sure to rule out other possibilities:
    Pancreatitis
    MI
    Pneumonia (all less likely if you see free air, so make sure to obtain an upright AXR)
    Esophagitis upright!
    Gastritis
    Gallbladder disease
    Aortic dissection

Physical Examination
    Check vital signs
    Look for peritoneal signs (guarding, rebound)
    Remember that findings are more subtle in the elderly and in patients on steroids

Diagnostic Tests
    Full laboratory panel including amylase/lipase
    Gastrin/calcium if there is suspicion of gastrinoma, hyperparathyroidism, or chronicity of problem
    For a perforated ulcer:
        Upright AXR
        Computed tomography (CT) scan (to demonstrate free air and rule out diverticulitis stenosis)
        CT or magnetic resonance imaging (MRI) of brain in symptomatic patients

M.A. Neff (ed.), *Passing the General Surgery Oral Board Exam*,
DOI 10.1007/978-1-4614-7663-4_13, © Springer Science+Business Media New York 2014

Magnetic resonance angiogram if available (if not, angiogram to include aortic arch and proximal common carotid artery)

For bleeding ulcer: Esophagogastroduodenoscopy (EGD) to rule out other pathology, help predict course, treat bleeding, and check for *H. pylori*

Treatment of bleeding ulcer by EGD:

Electrocautery

Heater probe

Injection therapy

Endoscopic appearance:

Clean-based ulcer (rarely rebleed)

Adherent clot (likely to rebleed)

Nonbleeding vessel (likely to rebleed)

For an obstruction, you need UG0049.

Treatment

For perforated ulcer:

There is no role for conservative treatment!

You need to initially resuscitate patient (intravenous fluids [IVF], antibiotics, H2 blockers).

Take to operating room (OR).

Make an upper midline incision.

Three choices:

1. High-risk patient (elderly, >24 h, unstable, advanced peritonitis):

Omental patch and abdominal lavage (>5 L saline)

2. Lower-risk patient (young, <24 h, stable, early peritonitis):

Omental patch, parietal cell vagotomy, lavage

3. Lower-risk patient with history of peptic ulcer disease (PUD):

Antrectomy (will include ulcer)/vagotomy, lavage

For bleeding ulcer:

Treatment initially is conservative with an EGD, transfusions, and H2 blockers.

You should know your limit of transfusions before going to the OR (>6 in 24 h or hemodynamic instability).

You should know what endoscopic appearance is a relative indication for surgery.

1. High-risk patient:

Perform vagotomy/pyloroplasty/oversew of ulcer (U stitch)

2. Lower-risk patient with small ulcer:

Oversew ulcer and perform parietal cell vagotomy

3. Lower-risk patient with large ulcer (> 2 cm) or history of PUD:

Perform antrectomy/vagotomy

For an obstruction:

Treatment is initially conservative with a trial of nasogastric tube (NGT) decompression and H2 blockers.

Check UGI series to confirm.

If this fails treatment (which it will on the boards), then proceed to the OR:

1. High-risk patient:

Gastrojejunostomy ± vagotomy

2. Low-risk patient:

Antrectomy and vagotomy (Billroth I reconstruction)

You should always try for a Billroth I (avoids afferent/efferent problems with the Billroth II and problems with a second anastomotic line). Be sure to extend at least 0.5 cm beyond the distal edge of the pylorus and check the proximal antrectomy line with a frozen section to show parietal cells.

If performing a pyloroplasty, you may not be able to do the typical Heineke-Mikulicz pyloroplasty with a scarred duodenum, so do a Finney or a Jaboulay (anastomosis involving distal stomach to the second portion of the duodenum). If all three are impossible, gastrojejunostomy is an effective emptying procedure.

Truncal vagotomy involves stripping the esophagus bare of areolar tissue in the distal 5–7 cm of esophagus.

If the patient has had prior surgery and preoperative workup reveals no specific cause for recurrence, take the next most aggressive option:

If there was a prior vagotomy with drainage, perform an antrectomy.

If there was a prior antrectomy with vagotomy, perform a subtotal gastrectomy.

Common Curveballs

EGD shows an adherent clot or visible vessel

Perforation is more than 24 h old

Perforation is in a patient with a long history of refractory ulcer disease

Perforation is in an elderly patient

Patient had prior abdominal surgery

You are not able to close the duodenal stump after antrectomy

Patient keeps requiring blood transfusions, but spread out over several days

Nonoperative treatment works but patient later presents with gastric outlet obstruction

Examiner asks you to describe how to perform a vagotomy/pyloroplasty/antrectomy and/or "U stitch" for bleeding duodenal ulcer

Gastrojejunostomy is complicated by a marginal ulcer, afferent loop syndrome, etc.

Duodenal stump leaks postoperatively

Patient rebleeds postoperatively after a U stitch was performed (consider angiographic embolization of gastroduodenal artery)

Patient has ZE syndrome

Patient had prior ulcer surgery

Clean Kills

Not ruling out other etiologies of epigastric pain

Trying to treat a perforated ulcer conservatively

Not trying to conservatively treat a bleeding ulcer at first presentation

Not being prepared to perform a different operation in someone with chronic symptoms

Not performing an EGD for a bleeding ulcer

Trying to treat gastric outlet obstruction with an endoscopic balloon dilatation

Performing any operation laparoscopically

Not knowing how to manage the difficult duodenal stump

Not knowing how to manage duodenal stump leak

Not oversewing the bleeding site when performing vagotomy/pyloroplasty

Not having an idea in your head about recurrence/mortality rates after different operations

Forgetting *H. pylori*

Trying to perform highly selective vagotomy in an unstable patient

Stats vary with the literature quoted, but rough rates are cited below:

	Recurrence (%)	Mortality (%)	Morbidity (%)
Vagotomy/pyloroplasty	10	1	15
Vagotomy/antrectomy	1	2	20
Parietal cell (highly selective) vagotomy	10	0	5

Summary

Duodenal pathology may present with bleeding, perforation, or obstruction. Surgical intervention is likely emergent with perforation, delayed with bleeding, and planned with obstructive pathology. The type of operative procedure performed should be dictated by both the presenting pathology as well as the patient's risk stratification. One should always biopsy the ulcer and consider *H. pylori* as an etiology.

Gastric Cancer

Concept

Gastric cancer will likely present as a large ulcer and biopsy-proven malignancy. The patient may not be candidate for anything but palliation. Be prepared to describe your workup and operation. Remember that gastric lymphoma is a different beast from gastric cancer.

Way Question May Be Asked?

"A 63 year-old man presents to the ED with UGI bleeding. After stabilization, an EGD is performed that reveals a large ulcer on the greater curvature. Biopsies return with well-differentiated adenocarcinoma. What do you do?"

The case may also present as a nonhealing ulcer, with pain, with perforation, with obstruction, or in work-up for melena or heme-positive stool.

How to Answer?

History
  Risk factors
  Weight loss
  Abdominal distension

Physical Examination
  Evidence of weight loss
  Palpable abdominal mass
  Prior surgical scars
  Lymphadenopathy (supraclavicular, periumbilical)
  Rectal examination (Blummer's shelf)

Diagnostic Tests
  Full laboratory panel
  UGI series
  EGD
  CT scan (to rule out metastatic disease)
  Can consider laparoscopy at outside of operation (to rule out liver metastases/carcinomatosis)
  Measure basal acid output (acchlorhydria associated with malignancy)

Location of Tumor

1. Tumors in antrum/distal third of stomach: radical subtotal gastrectomy involving 3 cm of the first part of the duodenum, hepatogastricomentum, greater omentum, and a D1 resection (immediately adjacent perigastric lymph nodes)
2. Tumors in corpus/middle third of stomach: subtotal or total gastrectomy depending on size of tumor
3. Tumors in proximal third of stomach: total gastrectomy, reconstruction with Roux-en-Y
4. Palliation → total gastrectomy (not gastroenterostomy!)

Comments on Surgery

Resect with 5-cm margins (if within 5 cm of gastroesophageal (GE) junction, perform a total gastrectomy).

Only resect the spleen if there is gross tumor involvement.

There is no evidence for resection of hepatic metastases.

Check the margins of resection by frozen section.

Perform en bloc resection of any directly invaded organ (spleen, tail of pancreas, kidney), except common bile duct or head of pancreas!

There is no evidence for Japanese-style D2 resection.

You should perform a D1 resection, which includes suprapyloric, infrapyloric, and nodes along the greater and lesser curvatures.

You can consider adjuvant and neoadjuvant treatments.

Do not forget vagotomy (anastomosis is an ulcer-producing procedure).

Do not forget the different types of reconstruction (Billroth II procedure if cancer).

Common Curveballs

Patient has a postoperative anastomotic bleed (especially if you did not perform vagotomy)

Patient has a postoperative leak

Patient is malnourished

Patient has a postoperative complication of gastric surgery:

Dumping syndrome—conservative measures first, then Roux-en-Y

Postvagotomy diarrhea—conservative measures first, then reversed jejunal segment

Alkaline reflux gastritis—confirm by hepatobiliary scan; conservative measures first, then Roux-en-Y gastrojejunostomy

Anastomotic bleed—EGD, then a suture ligation if EGD fails

Afferent loop syndrome—side-to-side jejunojejunostomy

Gastroperesis—conservative measures first, then a complete antrectomy or gastrectomy, depending on prior surgery, may be necessary

An ulcer that is high on the greater curve near the GE junction

Tumor penetrates into the surrounding structures (spleen, kidney, distal pancreas)

Examiner asks the difference between R1, R2, and R3 nodes

Pathology indicates a lymphoma

Patient actually has esophageal cancer and needs a traditional Ivor-Lewis resection

Patient presents later with evidence of metastatic disease/obstruction

Celiac node is positive (what does that mean?)

Patient has peritoneal metastases (how will you palliate patient?)

Examiner asks about treatment for duodenal stump leak (if early: duodenostomy, drains, nothing by mouth [NPO], total parenteral nutrition [TPN]); if late/abscess: CT-guided drain, NPO, TPN)

Clean Kills

Resecting hepatic metastases

Performing less than total gastrectomy for a tumor <5 cm from GE junction

Not staging the patient appropriately

Discussing laparoscopic resection of gastric cancer

Not checking the margins of resection by frozen section

Offering any therapy besides surgery for a "cure"

Discussing photodynamic therapy

Discussing endoscopic mucosal resections

Summary

Gastric cancer must be considered in the differential diagnosis when evaluating all gastric pathologies. A surgeon should be prepared to perform a cancer operation when operating on a patient with UGI bleeding and/or ulcer disease. Always take into consideration a patient's current and future nutrition status when planning the operation (i.e., placement of feeding jejunostomy).

Gastric Ulcer

Concept

The four basic types of gastric ulcers are categorized by location and etiology. Always have a high index of suspicion for malignancy and do everything possible to rule it out. The four types of gastric ulcers are:

I. Lesser curve, unrelated to acid

II. Gastric ulcer with associated duodenal ulcer, related to acid exposure

III. Prepyloric ulcer (within 3 cm of pylorus), related to acid exposure

IV. Adjacent to gastroesophageal junction (juxtacardial), unrelated to acid

Way Question May Be Asked?

"A 45-year-old man with a history of UGI bleeding had a gastric ulcer identified on EGD. He has been on omeprazole for 8 weeks and repeat EGD shows the ulcer is still present. What do you want to do?"

The question may go in the direction of how to initially treat this patient, how long to try acid suppressive therapy, and when to operate, or it may jump right into a discussion of how to manage a bleeding or perforated gastric ulcer. Size and pH are particularly important because most ulcers >3 cm and most ulcers in the achlorhydric patient will eventually need surgery.

How to Answer?

History
  Risk factors for PUD
  H. pylori treatment
  Steroid/NSAID use
  History of epigastric pain
  Iron-deficiency anemia
  Vomiting/bloating (from gastric outlet obstruction)
  Family history of ZE syndrome
  Use of antiulcer medications
  Relevant past medical history (heart disease, etc.)
  Prior surgeries (especially prior surgery for PUD)

Physical Examination
  Vital signs (tachycardia/hypotension to suspect shock)
  Abdominal examination (rigidity/peritoneal signs to suggest perforation)
  Rectal examination (heme positive, Blummer's shelf)

Diagnostic Studies
  Routine laboratory panels, including Type and Cross (T+C) and coagulation panel, especially if bleeding
  Electrolytes to show evidence of gastric outlet obstruction (low K, low Cl, high bicarbonate)
  Abdominal x-rays (to rule out free air)
  ± Barium UGI series
  Gastric acid analysis (achlorhydria is suggestive of cancer)
  EGD+biopsy (at least 10)
  Biopsy should include four quadrant margins, central biopsy, and brushings

Surgical Treatment

1. Resuscitate the unstable patient.
2. Repeat EGD/biopsy at 6–8 weeks for the chronic ulcer, treat medically, If improving, repeat EGD in 6–8 weeks:
   No improvement at first 6–8 week follow-up indicates surgery.
   Failure to disappear at second 6–8 week EGD indicates surgery.
3. Indications for surgery:
   Intractability
   Bleeding
   Perforation
   Obstruction
4. For type I (lesser curve) ulcer (most common):
   Antrectomy to include ulcer (goblet cells on duodenal side indicates adequate resection) and reconstruction with a Billroth I procedure. Make sure the frozen section is negative for malignancy before reconstructing with BI. Recurrence rate is 2 %.
5. For Type II and III ulcers:
   Antrectomy and truncalvagotomy
6. For Type IV ulcers:
   Resection with Roux-en-Y esophagogastrojejunostomy (Csendes' procedure)
7. For a bleeding ulcer:
   EGD+biopsy ± Angiogram with vasopressin/embolization
   Have a threshold in your mind of when to operate on patient (more than 6 U of packed red blood cells [pRBC] in 48 h—always consider baseline comorbidities in your limit)
   In the OR:
   (a) If the patient is stable, perform antrectomy to include the ulcer, and when possible, suture ligate ulcer, biopsy+antrectomy
   (b) If the patient is unstable, perform a wedge resection or suture/biopsy ulcer plus vagotomy/pyloroplasty
8. For a perforated ulcer:
   (a) If the patient is stable, perform an antrectomy to include the ulcer or antrectomy plus omental patch and biopsy the ulcer
   (b) If the patient is unstable, perform a biopsy and omental patch (a wedge resection of the ulcer is always an option if easy to do)

Common Curveballs

Biopsy comes back malignant, indeterminant, or benign
Type of ulcer (I–IV) switches during the scenario
Examiner asks your method to test for *H. pylori*
Patient fails medical management
Patient actually has gastric cancer (check frozen section before reconstruction)
Examiner asks your treatment algorithm for *H. pylori*
Examiner asks how to manage type IV ulcer intraoperatively
You are not able to encompass ulcer in antrectomy
Ulcer perforates
Patient bleeds postoperatively
Gastric acid measurements show achlorhydria
Examiner asks about postgastrectomy complications:
  Bleeding
  Dumping

Afferent/efferent obstruction
Postvagotomy diarrhea
Carcinoma

Clean Kills

Describing any laparoscopic approach
Not knowing how to deal with postgastrectomy syndromes
Not knowing how to describe your operation
Misdiagnosing a gastric cancer as a benign ulcer
Not testing for or treating *H. pylori*
Not knowing the importance of achlorhydria and its link to malignancy
Not rescoping/rebiopsying a patient with a chronic nonhealing ulcer
Not knowing the indications for surgery
Spending too long with angiographic methods to control bleeding
Not checking for malignancy before performing reconstruction (BII is preferred for malignant gastric ulcer)

Summary

A surgeon must be able to manage gastric ulcer disease in both the emergency department as well as the clinic. Questions can range from emergent operative management to outpatient treatment modalities. A firm grasp on the types and locations of the various gastric ulcers is important because this will dictate the operative procedure performed. Always biopsy the ulcer and be prepared for postgastrectomy complications.

Mallory-Weiss Tear

Concept

Mallory-Weiss tear presents as UGI bleeding in a patient after forceful vomiting. It is the result of a linear tear in the mucosa of the gastric cardia.

Way Question May Be Asked?

"A 23-year-old man presents to the ED with hematemesis after binge drinking."

Pain should not be a prominent feature; if it is, consider Boerhave's syndrome. This may be seen in patients with vomiting from other causes (pancreatitis, chemotherapy, etc.)

How to Answer?

Resuscitate the patient while doing history and physical examination!

History
    NSAID/ethanol use
    History of PUD
    H. pylori treatment
    Portal hypertension
    Hiatal hernia (tear is usually in gastric cardia rather than at the GE junction)
    Violent retching
        Remember your DDx of UGI bleeding: PUD, esophagitis, varices, Mallory–Weiss tear

Physical Examination
    Check vital signs
    Look for peritoneal signs (guarding, rebound)

Diagnostic Tests

Full laboratory panel, including coagulation factors, T+C

Management
    Place two large-bore intravenous (IV) lines and a large-caliber NGT.
    Irrigate via the NGT to estimate ongoing blood loss.
    Correct coagulation.
    Resuscitate the patient.
    Administer IV H2 blockers.
    Give a blood transfusion if the patient is unstable.
    Perform an EGD to identify and control bleeders.
        Rule out other pathology.
        Use a heater probe, sclerotherapy, electrocautery.
    Perform angiography to diagnose bleeder.
        Perform embolization of branches of left gastric.
        Give a selective infusion of vasopressin.
    Do not use Sengstaken–Blakemore tubes.

Surgery Indications
    Tranfusion of more than 6 U of PRBC
    Failure of EGD to stop bleeding
    Failure of angiographic embolization (used in patients with severe comorbidities)

Surgical Technique
    Make an upper midline incision.
    Explore UGI (may see subserosal hematoma at GE junction along the lesser curve of the stomach).
    Perform gastrostomy.

Oversew mucosal tear with absorbable, locking sutures.

Pack proximal and distal stomach with lap pads to locate the bleeding source.

Common Curveballs

EGD does not show mucosal laceration

Patient has evidence of perforation

Stomach is full of blood

EGD picks up other pathology

Endoscopic control/angiographic control fails

Patient has portal hypertension

Sclerotherapy results in esophageal perforation

Patient had prior abdominal surgery

Patient has tears in distal esophagus (may need left thoracotomy and esophagotomy and then suture ligation)

Patient may need to be intubated before EGD because of significant hematemesis (otherwise patient will aspirate)

Clean Kills

Jumping to angiography rather than EGD first

Using a Sengstaken-Blakemore tube

Not resuscitating the patient

Mistaking for Boerhave's syndrome

Performing any type of antiulcer surgery

Not looking for other pathology on EGD

Trying to do any of the above with a laparoscope

Summary

The majority of Mallory-Weiss tears are self-limiting. It is important to quickly stabilize and resuscitate the patient while taking a thorough history. Diagnostic modalities, such as EGD and angiography, may also be therapeutic in this setting. Surgery should be entertained if all other options have been exhausted or the patient is quickly deteriorating. In the operating room, the surgeon needs to be prepared to operate both below and above the diaphragm.

Upper Gastointestinal Bleeding

Concept

It is important to consider a broad DDx when consulted for upper gastrointestinal (GI) bleeding. Also pay close attention to the ABCs because a patient with massive hematemesis may exanguinate while you are still interviewing the patient. Perform a history with questions focused on the use of alcohol, recent vomiting, and a history of ulcer/liver disease.

Way Question May Be Asked?

"A 64 year-old woman presents to the ED with a chief complaint of weakness for 24 h and dark stools. She has a history of osteoarthritis currently being managed with NSAID therapy."

History is important because physical examination findings may be subtle. Coffee-ground emesis should serve to direct a practitioner toward the diagnosis through NGT lavage.

How to Answer?

<u>Take a brief history and physical examination while resuscitating the patient:</u>

History of PUD

Associated pain

Age

Aspirin, NSAID, dipyridamole, and steroid use

Current outpatient use of Coumadin, Plavix, Lovenox, or Pradaxa

Current outpatient use of antihypertensives or beta-blockers

Alcohol use

Recent retching/vomiting (Mallory-Weiss Tear)

Liver disease

Trauma/stress

History of UGI surgery (marginal ulcer)

History of abdominal aortic aneurysm (AAA) repair (aortoenteric fistula, initial small herald bleed followed a few days later with massive hemorrhage)

Physical Examination

Stigmata of liver disease (e.g., telangiectasia, jaundice, ascites)

Evidence of prior surgical scars

Melena or hematochezia on rectal examination

Bruit upon auscultation of the abdomen

Algorithm

ABCs ± endotracheal intubation depending on severity of bleed

Resuscitation (two large-bore IV lines, IVF, full laboratory panels including complete blood count, prothombin time/partial thromboplastin time, T+C, NGT)

Gastric lavage via NGT

Proton pump inhibitor (PPI) drip

Upper endoscopy if aspirate is bloody or clear (diagnostic and potentially therapeutic)

Tagged red blood cell scans

± Angiography

Surgery

Endoscopic methods to control bleeding
  Heater probe
  Electrocautery
  Epinephrine injection
  Mechanical occlusion via clips or band ligation/sclero-
  therapy (esophageal varices)
  (Appearance is important here because overlying clots/visi-
  ble vessels have a higher chance of rebreeding than a
  clean ulcer base.)

Angiography
  You can treat certain bleeds with intra-arterial gelfoam,
  metal coil springs, and vasopressin.
  It is useful for gastric/duodenal ulcers or Dieulafoy lesions.
  If bleeding successfully controlled, then initiate medical
  management.
  Administer PPI or H2 blockers and treat *H. pylori* if
  indicated.

Surgery
Surgery is reserved for unstable patients or patients with continued or recurrent bleeding (6 U pRBCs), complicated ulcer
disease, massive UGI bleeding, or nonhealing ulcers.
  For gastric neoplasms:
    If benign, perform a wedge resection (leiomyomas,
    hamartomas, hemangiomas, stromal tumors).
    If adenocarcinoma, resect with a 5–6 cm proximal
    margin (Billroth II). If adenocarcinoma is within
    5 cm of the GE junction, then perform a total
    gastrectomy.
  For stress gastritis, perform a total/near-total gastrectomy
  or gastric devascularization if unstable (quicker)
  For gastric ulcer:
    If patient is stable, perform a hemigastrectomy to
    include ulcer or wedge resection if ulcer is located
    proximal. Always send frozen section.
    If patient is unstable, perform a wedge resection and
    frozen section biopsy. Vagotomy and pyloroplasty
    can be considered in patients with a history of com-
    plicated ulcer disease.
  For a Dieulafoy lesion, perform a suture ligation or
  excision.
  For a duodenal ulcer:
    For high-risk/unstable patients, oversew the ulcer
    (U-stitch) and perform truncal vagotomy/
    pyloroplasty.
    For a stable patient with a small ulcer and no history of
    PUD, oversew the ulcer.
    For a stable patient with a small ulcer and history of
    PUD, oversew ulcer and perform a highly selective
    vagotomy.
    For a stable patient with a giant ulcer and history of
    PUD, perform an antrectomy plus vagotomy.

For bleeding from an anastomotic line from recent surgery, perform an EGD. If/when it fails, re-explore and
  ligate the bleeder.
For a Mallory-Weiss tear, perform an anterior gastrotomy
  and suture ligation of mucosal tears. If the tear is in the
  esophagus, perform a left thoracotomy/esophagotomy
  and suture ligate bleeders.
For hemosuccuspancreaticus, perform a distal pancreatectomy with excision of the pseudocyst and ligation
  of the splenic artery.
For an aorto-enteric fistula, control bleeding, resect the
  graft, close the enteric fistula site, and place a new
  extra-anatomic or in situ bypass graft.
For varices:
  If patient is a transplant candidate, perform a transjugular intrahepatic portosystemic shunt (TIPS) and
  then transplant when organ available.
  If patient is not a transplant candidate, perform emergency portacaval/splenorenal shunt or esophageal
  transection/suture ligation.
A four-port Minnesota tube may achieve hemostasis through
balloon tamponade prior to initiating surgical treatment.

Common Curveballs

Angiogram fails to localize lesion or embolization does not
  work
Endoscopy fails to localize lesion
Patient had prior ulcer surgery
Patient had prior AAA repair
Patient has coagulopathy
NGT lavage is not bilious
Bleeding is from the duodenum despite nonbloody, bilious
  NGT aspirate
Recurrent bleeding occurs after endoscopic treatment
Large ulcer is malignant
You may need to make gastrotomy/duodenotomy to localize
  bleeding
Bleeding is from nasopharynx or hemoptysis from lungs
Gastroenterologist is not available to perform EGD
Nonoperative therapy fails
"U-stitch" does not work (ligate gastroduodenal)

Clean Kills

Not placing NGT
Taking a prolonged history and physical examination
Improper resuscitation of patient
Not taking patient to surgery when appropriate
Not treating for *H. pylori*
Not taking biopsy of ulcer seen during EGD

Placing Sengstaken-Blakemore tube for Mallory-Weiss tear
Performing distal splenorenal shunt emergently for bleeding
  varices

Summary

To correctly diagnose and treat UGI bleeding, a multidisciplinary approach needs to be employed. A focused algorithm aimed at hemodynamic stabilization and localization via upper endoscopy is key to successful management. Upper endoscopy is potentially diagnostic and therapeutic and is indicated within 24 h of presentation, along with immediate initiation of intravenous infusion of a proton pump inhibitor. Surgical intervention may be required if the patient remains unstable or bleeding is refractory to all other treatment modalities.

Thoracic

Nicole M. Harris

Empyema

Concept

Empyema is an infection localized to the pleural space. It is often the result of a previous thin pleural effusion that has become thickened and exudative.

Way Question May Be Asked?

"A 55-year-old man in the intensive care unit [ICU] has persistent left loculated effusion. Thoracentesis is performed and reveals purulent material. What do you want to do?"

Differential Diagnosis

Pneumonia (streptococcal, pneumococcal, gram-negative, and anaerobic organisms are the most common pneumonias associated with empyema)

Esophageal perforation

Bronchopleural fistula

Recent surgery (chest or upper abdomen causing postoperative effusion)

Subphrenic abscess

Generalized sepsis

Undrained plueral effusion

Rupture of mediastinal or pulmonary abscess

Tuberculous empyema

How to Answer?

History

Tobacco use

Chest pain

Fever

Malaise

Loss of appetite

Weight loss

Cough or dyspnea (if underlying pneumonia is present)

Recent pneumonia or infection

History of cancer

Human immunodeficiency virus

Physical Examination

Auscultate chest

Examine for any adenopathy (cervical, axillary, clavicular)

If chest tube is present, evaluate output (color, consistency, change in output).

Diagnostic Studies

Chest x-ray (CXR) before thoracentesis/chest tube (posteroanterior/lateral):

Look for lesion, pneumonia, cavitary lesions

Look for air-fluid level (bronchopleural fistula)

CXR after thoracentesis/chest tube:

Confirm complete evacuation of effusion

Check for trapped lung, loculations, unexplained atelectasis (endobronchial lesion)

Confirm appropriate placement of chest tube

Send thoracentesis fluid for:

Cultures (aerobic, anaerobic, acid fast, fungal)

Cytology (to rule out malignancy)

Cell count, pH, lactate dehydrogenase, glucose

Computed tomography (CT) scan of chest to evaluate for:

Adenopathy (hilar, mediastinal, subcarinal)

Loculations

Mass lesion

Infiltrates

N.M. Harris, D.O., M.S. (✉)
General Surgery, University of Medicine and Dentistry of New Jersey, School of Osteopathic Medicine, Stratford, NJ, USA
e-mail: harrisn1@umdnj.edu

M.A. Neff (ed.), *Passing the General Surgery Oral Board Exam*, DOI 10.1007/978-1-4614-7663-4_14, © Springer Science+Business Media New York 2014

Pleural rind indicating trapped lung and reactive process
Air within the effusion indicating presence of infection
Bronchoscopy (if you suspect an endobronchial lesion)
Empyema stages:
Exudative: < 7 days
Fibropurulent: 7–14 days
Organized: > 14 days

Surgical Treatment

Complete and dependent drainage is required.
Exudative stage—Thoracentesis (usually prior to chest tube placement)
Chest tube (large caliber) drainage + antibiotics
Fibropurulent stage—Video-assisted thoracic surgery (VATS) exploration/pleurodesis (pleural biopsy/cytology if suspect malignancy) or limited thoracotomy
Organized stage—VATS decortication
Thoracotomy open decortication
Rib resection and Eloesser flap (skin sutured to parietal pleura) is used in a high-risk patient!

Common Curveballs

Cytology is positive for malignancy (switch scenarios to workup for malignancy depending on what pathology demonstrates as primary)
Empyema fails treatment with chest tube (perform VATS or thoracotomy)
Patient develops bronchopleural fistula after thoracotomy (following lobectomy or pneumonectomy)
Patient requires evaluation of cause of fistula, drainage, and obliteration of pleural space
Stains for acid-fast bacilli are positive
Lung does not reexpand after drainage of effusion/empyema (requires decortication via VATS or thoracotomy with pleuradesis)
Empyema is the result of some extrapulmonary process (perforated esophagus, subphrenic abscess, etc.—scenario switch!)

Clean Kills

Forgetting pulmonary function tests (PFTs) if proceeding towards thoracotomy
Describing VATS as an option if you do not do (or know how to do) this procedure
Mentioning an Eloesser flap if you do not know how to perform it or know its indications (reserved for high-risk patients or in chronic empyema with residual pleural space)

Not checking cytology on drained effusion
Not performing bronchoscopy for persistently unexpanded lung fields

Summary

The keys to empyema are to identify early, isolate organisms, and begin empiric antibiotic treatment as soon as possible (streptococcal, pneumococcal, gram-negative, and anaerobic organisms). Suspect empyema if pleural effusion has air in it. Remember your stages and what surgical procedure is appropriate for each stage. Ultimately, drainage is the end goal.

Lung Cancer

Concept

Surgical treatment is the only potential cure for lung cancer. The key is to determine if the patient is resectable or not (by preoperative PFTs and cardiac evaluation). It may present as a solitary pulmonary nodule (for which only 1 in 20 turns out to actually be malignant) or multiple nodules.

Way Question May Be Asked?

"A 64-year-old woman is found to have a new lesion ~2 cm in diameter in the left upper lobe. It was found on a preoperative chest x-ray prior to a hysterectomy for fibroids. What do you want to do?"

How to Answer?

History
50–60 years old
Tobacco use (how long and how much)
Asbestos/arsenic/chromium/nickel exposure
Chemical exposure (previous work environments is important)
Travel history
History of prior cancer (metastatic vs. recurrence?)
Significant secondhand smoke exposure
Radiation exposure

Common Symptoms
New voice changes/neurologic symptoms
Weight loss
Chest/bone pain
Shortness of breath

Hemoptysis/obstructive pneumonia

Symptoms of syndrome of inappropriate antidiuretic hormone secretion

Physical Examination

Auscultate chest

Examine for any adenopathy (clavicular, axillary, and cervical)

Palpate liver

Diagnostic Studies

CXR, compared to prior CXR (if <3 cm, present on prior CXR, and unchanged, you can follow)

CT scan (chest/abdomen/pelvis)

   Evaluate mass size and location

   Evaluate for metastases

   Evaluate lymph nodes (mediastinal, hilar, subcarinal, aortic, clavicular)

   If it is a solitary nodule and calcified or radiologically stable by CT for 2 years, it is less likely to be malignant

Morning sputum cytologies and cultures (three)

Flexible bronchoscopy and potential biopsy (if proximal lesion)

Biopsy of lesion (bronchscopy if centrally located lesion, interventional radiology biopsy if peripherally located lesion)

   Brush Biopsy

   Transbronchial

   Percutaneous by CT

If there is mediastinal lymphadenopathy and a lung lesion, you can perform mediastinoscopy or obtain mediastinal biopsy (will achieve both tissue diagnosis and help stage disease)

Need preoperative pulmonary tests:

   Arterial blood gas

      PFTs (>80 % predicted for FEV1 or Diffusing capacity of the lung for carbon monoxide (DLCO), predictor of successful outcome)

      Ventilation/perfusion scan (to predict postoperative FEV1)

      May require PET-CT for evaluation of metastases

Staging of Lung Cancer

Tx: primary tumor cannot be assessed or malignant cells are present on bronchial washings but not appreciated on CT

T0: no evidence of primary tumor

Tis: carcinoma in situ

T1a: ≤2 cm, no invasion of lobar bronchus

T1b: ≥2–3 cm, no invasion of lobar bronchus

T2a: ≥3–5 cm, or main bronchus >2 cm from carina, or atelectasis or obstructive pneumonitis to hilum (not entire lung), or invasion visceral pleura

T2b: >5–7 cm, or main bronchus >2 cm from carina, or atelectasis or obstructive pneumonitis to hilum (not entire lung), or invasion of visceral pleura

T3: >7 cm, <2 cm from carina, atelectasis of whole lung, tumor invading chest wall, diaphragm, or mediastinal pleura, phrenic nerve, parietal pericardium, or nodules in same lung

T4: Tumor in carina, tumor invades any mediastinal structure (esophagus, heart, great vessels, trachea, spine) or satellite tumor nodules within ipsilateral lobe, or malignant pleural/pericardial effusion

N1: ipsilateral peribronchial and/or ipsilateral hilar lymph nodes and intrapulmonary nodes

N2: ipsilateral mediastinal and/or subcarinal lymph nodes

N3: contralateral mediastinal nodes, contralateral hilum, ipsilateral or contralateral scalene/supraclavicular nodes involved

Mx: metastasis not evaluated

M0: no distant metastases

M1a: separate tumor nodule(s) in a contralateral lobe or tumor with pleural nodules or malignant pleural or pericardial effusion

M1b: distant metastasis

Stages of Lung Cancer:

Stage IA	T1a–T1b	N0	M0
Stage IB	T2a	N0	M0
Stage IIA	T1a,T1b,T2a	N1	M0
	T2b	N0	M0
Stage IIB	T2b	N1	M0
	T3	N0	M0
Stage IIIA	T1a, T1b, T2a, T2b	N2	M0
	T3	N1, N2	M0
	T4	N0, N1	M0
Stage IIIB	T4	N2	M0
	Any T	N3	M0
Stage IV	Any T	Any N	M1a or M1b

Contraindications to Surgical Resection

   Stage III and greater

   Predicted postoperative FEV1 or DLCO <40 %

Surgical Procedures

   Mediastinoscopy for mediastinal/hilar/subcarinal nodules/lympadenopathy

Chamberlain procedure for right-sided nodules and enlarged left paratracheal nodes

Lobectomy via VATS or thoracotomy

En bloc resection if there is chest wall involvement

Pneumonectomy (if there is a hilar lesion, the lesion encompasses all lobes on a given side [crosses fissures])

Common Curveballs

No lesion is benign (even if on prior CXR)

Lesion is metastatic disease (scenario switch—will you perform pulmonary metastatectomy?)

Criteria for resection

1. Pulmonary metastases appear to be completely resectable on CT
2. Adequate cardiopulmonary reserve to undergo resection
3. Technical feasibility of operation
4. Contolled primary tumor site
5. Absence of extrapulmonary metastatic disease
6. Resection of one or more lung lesions if a new primary lung cancer cannot be excluded, there is symptomatic metastases, or tissue is needed for a novel approach or clinical trial

Colorectal cancer is the only cancer for which there are guidelines for pulmonary metastases resection. However, potential for long-term improvement in 5-year survival rates have been predicted in soft tissue sarcoma, renal cell, germ cell, gynecological, melanoma, head and neck, osteosarcoma, breast, hepatocellular, and gastric cancers—each with their own set of slightly variable indications and preoperative workup and evaluation.

Tumor has characteristics of unresectability

Patient has Horner's syndrome (miosis, ptosis, and anhidrosis; lung lesion likely at apex)

Patient has positive cytology from pleural effusion (already stage IV; no surgical resection)

Patient has positive cervical lymph nodes (Stage IIIB; no surgical resection)

Patient has tracheoesophageal fistula

Patient has recurrent laryngeal nerve or phrenic nerve paralysis

Presents as hemoptysis (25–50%; attempt bronchoscopy for proximal lesion)

Presents as pleural effusion (unresectable)

Presents as lung abscess

Tumor is hormonally active

Adrenocorticotropic hormone (ACTH) (causes Cushing's syndrome, common with small cell lung cancer [SCLC] and carcinoid)

Parathyroid hormone (PTH)-like (causes hypercalcemia, most common with SCLC)

Antidiuretic hormone (ADH) (causes hyponatremia, often in SCLC)

Patient has post-pneumonectomy

Patient has bronchopleural fistula (When this occurs within 1 week of surgery, there is likely no empyema. If it occurs >2 weeks postoperatively, it is likely empyema. Signs include fever, productive cough, hemoptysis, subcutaneous emphysema, and persistent air leak from a chest tube. Treatment is drainage of the pleural space, systemic antibiotics, and then repair of the air leak once the postpneumonic space has been sterilized.)

Patient has atrial fibrillation (most common postpneumonectomy arrhythmia; treat with amiodarone)

Patient has mediastinal shift in the recovery room (Rule out contralateral pneumothorax by CXR. If present, evacuate air by decompression and chest tube. If acute hemothorax is suspected, proceed with surgical re-exploration and control of bleeding sources.)

Clean Kills

Forgetting PFTs prior to thoracotomy

Describing VATS or segmentectomy or wedge resection as an option if you do not do (or know how to do) this procedure

Not performing bronchoscopy

Not checking prior CXR

Operating on small cell carcinoma

Not performing mediastinoscopy preoperatively when indicated

Offering palliative resections

Not knowing the staging system

Summary

Evaluation and treatment of lung cancer is guided by preoperative workup and staging. It is imperative to perform preoperative PFTs and know which stages of lung cancer surgical resection are not indicated. Treatment is often a multidisciplinary approach between the pulmonologist, medical oncologist, and surgeon. A detailed and extensive preoperative workup is key in lung cancer.

Trauma and Critical Care

Leigh Ann Slater, Luis J. Garcia, Thomas Cartolano,
Catherine Garrison Velopulos, Farshad Farnejad,
and Elliott R. Haut

Abdominal Compartment Syndrome

Concept

Abdominal compartment syndrome (ACS) is similar to other compartment syndromes in that it occurs when the pressure inside a closed compartment (i.e., the abdomen) becomes elevated and affects the normal function of the contents of that compartment. ACS is defined as a sustained intra-abdominal pressure (IAP) >20 mm Hg that is associated with new organ dysfunction/failure.

Elevated IAP has a direct effect on nearly every body system, including the pulmonary, cardiovascular, renal, neurologic, and gastrointestinal (GI) systems.

Way Question May Be Asked?

"You are called to see a 75-year-old man in the intensive care unit (ICU) 5 h after a sigmoid colectomy with end colostomy for diverticulitis that was performed by your senior partner, who just left on vacation. The patient is now hypotensive with a decreasing urine output. What do you want to do?"

L.A. Slater, M.D. (✉) • Luis J. Garcia, M.D.
Catherine Garrison Velopulos, M.D. • Farshad Farnejad, M.D., M.P.H.
Elliott R. Haut, M.D., F.A.C.S.
Department of Surgery, Division of Acute Care Surgery,
The Johns Hopkins University School of Medicine, Baltimore,
MD 21287, USA
e-mail: lslater2@jhmi.edu

T. Cartolano, D.O.
General Surgery, University of Medicine and Dentistry of
New Jersey, School of Osteopathic Medicine, Stratford, NJ, USA

In an alternate presenting scenario, you may be called to see a patient because of high ventilatory pressures, for whom you have to rule out many causes (acute respiratory distress syndrome, pneumothorax [PTX], mucus plug) before diagnosing ACS.

How to Answer?

You have to use a systematic approach when faced with a patient with oliguria.

Is It Pre-Renal?
   Shock/hemorrhage/sepsis/long operation/underresuscitation
   Cardiogenic shock? Pump failure? Acute myocardial infarction (MI)/congestive heart failure (CHF)
      Vascular etiology? Embolic after suprarenal aortic clamp
Is It Intra-Renal?
Acute tubular necrosis from any hypotension (perioperatively)
Nephrotoxic medications
   Is It Post-Renal/Obstructive?
      Ureteral occlusion/injury
      Foley catheter is kinked, clogged, clotted, etc.
The following should be mentioned in your answer:
   Brief history and physical examination (although your patient in the scenario will likely be on a ventilator)
Assess volume status (central venous pressure [CVP], Swan, echocardiography [echo])
Baseline renal function/trend in perioperative urine output—is it acute onset oliguria?
Perioperative events—large-volume resuscitation/transfusions?
Hypotension? Line placed in operating room (OR) causing pneumothorax?
   Review medications that are potentially toxic to kidneys.
   Is the Foley catheter patent?

Briefly mentioning the above possibilities will let the examiner know that you have a broad differential and are not blindly jumping to the obvious diagnosis.

Diagnosis is made by confirming elevated IAP. Have very low threshold to check bladder pressure. Some suggest routine monitoring of IAP in all patients in the ICU with any organ dysfunction.

Treatment

Always consider nonoperative possibilities before immediately jumping to surgical decompression. Options include catheter drainage of abdominal fluid/ascites, decompression of GI tract (nasogastric tube (NGT), rectal tube), and paralysis. If there is no rapid or immediate improvement, you should move to prompt surgical decompression. You will need to leave the abdomen open (see Damage Control Surgery section for options for temporary closure).

Common Curveballs

Examiner tries to lead you away from fluid resuscitation by emphasizing the multiple liters of IVF already given intraoperatively (remember insensible loses up to 1 L hour in the OR with abdomen open and the bowel prep put the patient behind from fluid standpoint before surgery)

Patient has a history of renal insufficiency, MI, or only has one kidney

Nothing you do works (the examiner is just testing your thinking—make sure you follow laboratory tests)

Patient has electrolyte abnormalities, especially potassium (change any medications that need renal dosing and consider need for dialysis)

Clean Kills

Not ruling out compartment syndrome (check bladder pressures)

Not looking for other causes of renal failure (it will be whatever you leave out)

Not assessing volume status (CVP or Swan or echo)

Not ruling out a pneumothorax, MI, or pulmonary embolism (PE) as the cause of hypotension

Not ruling out PTX, mucus plug, or endotracheal tube kink as cause of high airway pressures

Not checking the Foley catheter (is it kinked?)

Diurese with no objective assessment of volume status

Not reassessing the patient frequently (laboratory tests/physical examination)

Summary

ACS can be manifest in many ways:
1. **Pulmonary compliance suffers as pulmonary vascular resistance increases as a result of increased intra-thoracic pressures. This presents as elevated airway pressures and/or decreased ventilator volumes.**
2. **Reduction in cardiac output and/or systolic blood pressure is a result of decreased venous return from direct compression of the inferior vena cava (IVC) and portal vein. Increased intrathoracic pressure also results in reduced IVC/superior vena cava flow.**
3. **Elevations in IAP are associated with incremental reductions in measured renal plasma flow and glomerular filtration rate. This results in a decline in urine output, beginning with oliguria.**
4. **High intra-thoracic pressure can lead to impaired venous return from the brain and may lead to elevated intra-cranial pressures, which can be detrimental, especially in the multiply injured trauma patient.**

Colon and Rectal Trauma

Concept

Colon and rectal trauma is likely to be seen in the context of multiple other injuries. Typical examples are a gunshot wound (GSW) to the abdomen with small bowel and colon injury or a fall with a pelvic fracture and obvious rectal injury.

Way Question May Be Asked?

"A 36-year-old man is being evaluated for a pelvic fracture in the emergency department (ED) and, on rectal examination, there is gross blood. What do you want to do?"

This question may also be asked in the setting of a blunt trauma patient with a pelvic fracture or in the setting of a GSW to the abdomen, pelvis, or thigh. Less likely, the scenario will be from direct rectal trauma or a foreign body. Again, always remember to deal with life-threatening injuries first.

How to Answer?

Start out the same was as for every trauma patient—a brief AMPLE history while resuscitating:

ABCs:

Airway and C-spine control (intubate with collar on)

Breathing

Circulation, intravenous (IV) access

Disability (neurologic status)

Exposure

AMPLE History:

Allergies

Medications

Past medical/surgical history

Last meal

Events

Resuscitation (IVF, full laboratory tests including prothrombin time (PT)/partial thromboplastin time (PTT), T+C, NGT, Foley)

Secondary Survey:

Head-to-toe physical examintion when primary survey is complete and patient stabilized

Do not skip the secondary survey or you will miss an injury

Rectal examination for injury, motor tone, blood, "high riding prostate" (sign of possible urethral injury—goes along with blood at penile meatus and scrotal hematoma)

May need rigid proctocope/sigmoidoscope

Do not forget to immobilize and stabilize the pelvic fracture!

Chest and pelvis x-ray in trauma bay

Stable patient may receive computed tomography (CT) scan

Unstable patient gets focused assessment with sonography for trauma (FAST) or diagnostic peritoneal lavage (DPL) in the trauma bay; if positive, proceed to OR for exploratory laparotomy

Surgical Treatment

Resuscitate the patient

Rule out other life-threatening injuries

Colon injuries:

1. Primary repair is a reasonable option for many patients—must meet all of these criteria

Hemodynamically stable

Small laceration (<1 cm)

Contamination minimal

Not delayed presentation

No other major abdominal injuries

Not getting massive blood transfusion

Debride back to healthy tissue

Close in one or two layers

2. Resection and anastomosis can be considered—best for patients with most of above criteria (i.e., not too sick) but in whom you cannot simply close the hole primarily

Sometimes consider proximal diverting loop (i.e., ielostomy), which is easier to take down later but protects anastamosis while it heals

3. Hartman's/colostomy is a better option for the following:

Patients in shock

Multiple other injuries

Destructive wounds

Gross contamination

Rectal injuries:

Intraperitoneal rectal injuries are treated the same as colon injuries

Extraperitoneal rectal injuries

Repair and diverting stoma (sigmoid loop colostomy)

Consider presacral drainage (although done less frequently these days)

3-cm curvilinear incision between coccyx and rectum

Posterior dissection carried up to level of injury

Place two Penrose drains

Distal rectal washout

2 L of irrigant following an anal stretch

Common Curveballs

Patient has other associated injuries (intra- and extra-abdominal)

Patient has a missed bowel injury

Examiner asks you to describe the treatment for rectal injury

Patient is unstable intraoperatively (can do damage control, leave colon in discontinuity and continue at next operation)

Patient develops abdominal compartment syndrome postoperatively

Patient has a leak after primary repair of colon wound

Patient has an open pelvic fracture (gets diverting sigmoid colostomy regardless of whether rectal injury or not)

Patient with pelvic fracture has a coincident bladder injury (always divert fecal stream if there is another injury, such as bladder/urethra)

Clean Kills

Not knowing it is preferable to primarily repair most colon injuries

Not knowing how to treat rectal injury with diversion, drains, and washout

Not looking for other injuries

Not looking for rectal or bladder injury in pelvic fracture

Summary

Always follow the standard trauma algorithm to avoid missing an injury. Identify and treat life-threatening injuries first and in a timely manner before launching into the details of your operative management.

Compartment Syndrome

Concept

Elevated pressure in a closed compartment leads to ischemic damage to muscle and nerve, which may lead to limb loss and myoglobinuria with resulting renal failure. This occurs most commonly in the extremities as the result of crush injuries, vascular injuries, reperfusion after prolonged ischemia, compression by cast, or burns. The key is maintaining a high index of suspicion.

Way Question May Be Asked?

"You have just finished repairing a GSW to the femoral artery and vein and you notice that it took you about 6 h to perform. The nurse wants to know if there is anything else you would like to do."

Rarely would the question be so leading, but remember compartment syndrome in any case of vascular trauma, orthopedic trauma, or vascular repair. Also, consider the diagnosis in patients with deep burns to the extremity.

How to Answer?

History
   Mechanism of injury
   Pain out of proportion to injury
   Pain distal from site of injury
   Tingling/numbness in extremity
Physical Examination
   Tense, swollen extremity
   Pain with passive range of motion
   Sensory deficit
   Absence of pulses is <u>late</u> finding
   In the leg, examine:
      1. Sensation in first web space (deep peroneal nerve = anterior compartment)
      2. Sensation of dorsum of foot (superficial peroneal nerve = lateral compartment)
      3. Sensation of plantar surface (tibial nerve = deep posterior compartment)
      4. Pain with passive dorsiflexion and plantar flexion of great toe
Diagnostic Tests
   Measuring compartment pressures
      1. Use specific device, such as a solid-state transducer intracompartmental catheter
      2. Attach a 16-g needle to an A-line setup with three-way stopcock. Using sterile saline, zero monitor, and inject 1 cc into the compartment.
   Should measure all compartments at risk
   Show measure and repeat examination at intervals if suspicious

Surgical Treatment

Decompression for:
   Strong clinical suspicion
   Compartment pressure > 40 mm Hg
   Compartment pressure within 30 mm Hg of diastolic blood pressure (BP)
Bivalve any cast
OR for fasciotomy
   In leg:
      Make two incisions.
      The first incision is from the knee to ankle and centered between the anterior and lateral compartments.
      Divide the fascia 1 cm above and below the intermuscular septum to free the anterior and lateral compartments, respectively.
      Be careful to avoid the superficial peroneal nerve in the lateral compartment.
      The second incision is also from the knee to ankle and is 2 cm posterior to the posteromedial border of the tibia.
      Avoid the saphenous vein.
      Divide the fascia overlying gastrocnemius and soleus muscles (medial compartment).
      Detach the soleus from the posterior tibia to reach the fascia of the deep compartment and incise.
Apply loose dressings.
Keep the extremity at heart level. (Do not raise!)
Return to the OR ever 36 h to debride necrotic tissue and change dressings.
Keep the patient well hydrated to avoid renal failure.
Perform a split-thickness skin graft if you cannot close after 7 days.

Common Curveballs

Patient has altered sensorium/is intubated and you cannot obtain history and physical examination

Compartment pressure is 30 mm Hg

Compartment pressure changes on repeated recordings

Examiner asks you to describe how to perform a fasciotomy

Patient has necrotic muscle after the fasciotomy and examiner asks if you want to debride (no, wait and return to the OR; necrotic tissue may improve)

Patient develops myoglobinuria and renal failure

Clean Kills

Not correctly diagnosing compartment syndrome

Only performing escharotomies when fasciotomy is indicated

Not being able to describe a fasciotomy

Waiting until extremity is pulseless before performing fasciotomy

Trying to describe a one-incision quadruple fasciotomy for the leg

Summary

Compartment syndrome can have a devastating effect on a patient who suffers limb injury. A common cause is secondary to reperfusion injury after prolonged ischemia. Once the diagnosis has been made, immediate decompression is warranted. Lower extremity fasciotomies are performed through a two-incision approach (medial and lateral). Upper extremity fasciotomies should be performed with volar and radial incisions. Prophylactic fasciotomy for high-risk patients should be considered after prolonged ischemic time.

Duodenal Trauma

Concept

Duodenal trauma is a rare isolated injury. It is highly associated with injury to adjacent structures, including the pancreas and pancreatic duct, common bile duct, aorta, inferior vena cava, and/or superior mesenteric artery. The diagnosis is most often made intraoperatively. The classic scenario for a blunt case is a child or teenager with a duodenal hematoma after blunt abdominal trauma such, as a fall forward onto bicycle handlebars. A classic case for an adult is a gunshot wound.

Way Question May Be Asked?

"You are exploring a patient for a splenic laceration and find a periduodenal hematoma on your exploratory laparotomy. What do you want to do?"

You may also be given the diagnosis of duodenal hematoma on CT scan after blunt trauma with history of a patient receiving a blow to the epigastrium. It could also be a straightforward diagnosis of a hole in the duodenum after an abdominal gunshot wound.

How to Answer?

Basically, this is more of a management question rather than a diagnosis question. Quickly conduct a basic trauma evaluation with ABCs, look for other injuries, and resuscitate. But, in this case the examiner wants to hear how you operate to fix this injury.

Nonoperative Management

Preoperatively diagnosed duodenal trauma (duodenal hematoma) may be treated without immediate surgical intervention. This needs to be an isolated duodenal hematoma—most likely seen on CT scan and then confirmed by gastrograffin followed by barium swallow studies that show narrowing of the duodenal lumen without evidence of leak/extravasation. Patient is admitted, kept NPO, and observed with nasogastric suction and IV nutrition. Observation is limited to 4 weeks for a duodenal wall hematoma, at which time you should consider exploration of the patient who is not improving.

Surgical Treatment

1. The first step is to explore/expose intraoperatively to identify or rule out injury to pancreas and adjacent ductal and major vascular structures (i.e., portal vein, vena cava, superior mesenteric artery)
    (a) Extended Kocher maneuver from porta hepatis to superior mesenteric vessels to visualize the entire posterior duodenum
    (b) You can perform an extended mobilization from the left side as well to divide the ligament of Treitz in order to see D3/D4
    (c) You may also need to add the Cattell-Braasch maneuver (mobilize the entire right colon up out of the retroperitoneum—good to look at the ureter, vena cava, right kidney) to look at other structures on right side
2. In the operating room, fully expose the duodenum and determine amount of tissue loss and location of injury (D1 versus D4, etc.), as well as type and severity of other injuries (i.e., liver, spleen, colon, ureter)

(a) Intramural hematoma: if preoperatively diagnosed, you can observe. But once in the OR, you need to explore and rule out a full-thickness laceration or leak

(b) Simple laceration: primary repair—a one- or two-layer closure (transversely so you do not narrow the lumen) ± omental patch

(c) More complicated lacerations: debridement and primary closure, as long as there is no luminal compromise or tension, with an omental patch

(d) Large laceration to the second portion of the duodenum or whenever you are unable to do a primary repair: Roux-en-Y reconstruction

(e) Multiple complex lacerations: pyloric exclusion
   Pyloric closure (staple from outside or sew from inside)
   Gastrojejunostomy
   Primary repair of duodenal lacerations

(f) Always leave drains in every duodenal repair case

(g) Always decompress with a nasogastric tube from above. You can also use a nasoduodenal tube through the pylorus to decompress the duodenum. This is better than older approach of tube duodenosotmy.

(h) If there is associated contusion to the head of the pancreas, you must consider looking for the common bile duct (CBD) and/or pancreatic duct injury. Do not open an uninjured CBD or uninjured duodenum to perform a cholangiogram. You can do a cholangiogram by accessing gallbladder (then removing) if very concerned.

(i) Avoid temptation to perform the "trauma Whipple." Only perform if you have no other safe choice. This is mostly appropriate if it was basically already done by the injury. Consider "damage control" and reconstructing at a later date.

(j) Consider a feeding surgical jejunostomy tube or nasojejunal tube placed at time of surgery to allow early enteral feeding.

Common Curveballs

Patient has multiple other injuries (may be abdominal or outside abdomen)

Patient has pancreatic injury (i.e., combined pancreaticoduodenal)

Patient becomes acidotic and coagulopathic intraoperatively (you should perform "damage control" surgery)

Patient fails nonoperative management (you can go to surgery in a delayed fashion)

Patient has a postoperative leak

Patient has postoperative fever—look for leak, abscess

Examiner asks about your postoperative management (gastrograffin GI study, drains, feeding)

Clean Kills

Not looking for associated injuries (especially pancreas)

Not adequately fully visualizing duodenum (need to be able to describe intraoperative techniques)

Not being familiar with the various ways to surgically manage duodenal injury

Not placing a nasogastric tube and external drain

Not using damage control techniques for an unstable, cold, coagulopathic, acidotic patient (detailed examination of the pancreas should await a second look in this scenario)

Summary

Always follow the standard trauma algorithm to avoid missing an injury. Identify and treat life-threatening injuries first and in a timely manner before launching into details of your operative management. Be familiar with several different methods of duodenal repair based on the location and severity of the injury, and always leave a nasogastric tube and external drain. Consider distal feeding access (can be a nasojejunal tube) when prolonged NPO status is anticipated. Remember to use damage control techniques in the cold, coagulopathic, acidotic patient in extremis. Definitive reconstruction of pancreatic injuries must wait in this setting.

Genitourinary Trauma

Concept

Genitourinary (GU) trauma will usually be couched in another question, such as the multiply injured trauma patient who has a retroperitoneal hematoma seen after exploration of a penetrating abdominal injury. It may also be seen in the setting of blunt trauma with a pelvic fracture. Do not forget the priorities in trauma patients (ABCs).

Way Question May Be Asked?

"A 19-year-old man is seen in the emergency room after a GSW to his right flank with a systolic BP of 90 and gross hematuria after placement of a Foley catheter. What do you want to do?"

The question could also have presentation after a fall from a height or a car accident with a pelvic fracture secondary to blunt trauma. Make a decision on the stability of the patient early and frequently reassess throughout the scenario.

How to Answer?

ABCs
Primary survey
Secondary survey
History
    AMPLE history (Mechanism of injury, etc.)
    Pre-existing renal disease
Physical Examination
    Full examination in secondary survey especially
        Blood at urethral meatus
        Stool guiac for possible rectal injury
        High-riding prostate in males
Diagnostic Testing
    Need complete laboratory panels, chest x-ray (CXR), urinalysis (hematuria)
    DPL in unstable patients (this is a common board theme!)
    CT scan in stable patients with IV contrast (evaluate both kidneys)
    Retrograde cystourethrogram to define urethral injury

Surgical Treatment

Be sure to rule out other intra/extra-abdominal injuries
1. Bladder injuries
    (a) Extraperitoneal female—Foley catheter or suprapubic cystostomy
    (b) Extraperitoneal male—suprapubic cystostomy
    (c) Intraperitoneal—primary repair and suprapubic cystostomy
2. Ureteral injuries—key is level of injury
    (a) Lower third—ureterneocystostomy ± psoas hitch
    (b) Middle third—end-to-side ureteroureterostomy to other ureter (most urologists hate this option)
    (c) Proximal third—nephrostomy tube in ipsilateral kidney
    (d) If tissue loss minimal, you can try primary repair over a stent
    Always drain the site of repair!
3. Renal parenchymal injury
    (a) Nonvisualization on CT or intravenous pyelogram—angiography and/or exploration promptly (1 h warm ischemia time is too much!)
    (b) Renal vein injury—repair in stable patients, otherwise ligate
    (c) Renal artery—repair in stable patients, otherwise nephrectomy
    (d) Extravasation—repair or partial resection in stable patient, otherwise nephrectomy
    (e) Pedicle avulsion—nephrectomy

4. Retroperitoneal hemotomas
    (a) All hematomas in penetrating trauma should be explored unless subhepatic
    (b) Can observe hematoma in blunt trauma as long as not expanding
    (c) Should explore central, portal, and pericolonic hematomas
5. Urethral injuries
    Whether partial or total, gets cystostomy and *delayed* urethroplasty
6. To expose retroperitoneal structures
    Mattox maneuver on left
    Cattell maneuver on right

Common Curveballs

Patient is unstable
Patient has intraoperative retroperitoneal hematoma
Patient has one kidney
Patient has bladder injury (first extra-peritoneal, then intraperitoneal)
Patient has ureteral injury in a variety of locations
Patient has postoperative hypertension from activation of the renin/angiotensin/aldosterone axis
Patient has postoperative extravasation of contrast from a bladder or kidney injury
Examiner asks when you will perform a "trauma nephrectomy"
Patient has injury to other retroperitoneal organs (duodenum, pancreas, colon)
Examiner asks you to describe performing a psoas hitch or nephrostomy tube placement

Clean Kills

Any sort of laparoscopic treatment/evaluation
Getting stuck on therapeutic embolization for renal laceration
Not checking the meatus/rectum in a pelvic fracture patient
Not exploring retroperitoneal hematoma when appropriate
Not performing nephrectomy when appropriate
Not ruling out other, more life-threatening injuries
Not looking for injuries to other retroperitoneal organs
Performing a CT scan in an unstable patient

Summary

Injury to the genitourinary tract is a common occurrence after both blunt and penetrating trauma. Delayed recognition

of these injuries may have the unique complication of urinary extravasation. To avoid the subsequent morbidity, a high index of suspicion must be maintained and the appropriate radiographic evaluation performed. The indications, timing, and method of diagnostic imaging performed in patients with suspected urinary tract injury have been controversial. Additionally, improved imaging techniques have led to re-evaluation of the methods of diagnosing potential urinary tract injury. When multiple injuries coexist in a patient with GU trauma, injuries to the GU tract must be assessed as to their contribution to the immediate life-threatening situations.

Liver Trauma

Concept

The liver is one of the most frequently injured abdominal organs. Remember to resuscitate the patient and rule out other injuries. Perform nonoperative management in a stable patient with no other indications for abdominal exploration.

Way Question May Be Asked?

"You are called to the trauma bay to evaluate a 26-year-old motorcyclist injured after impact against a guard rail. He is tachycardic, hypotensive, and has contusions about the right side of his chest and abdomen. What do you want to do?"

You may also be given the intraoperative setting of multiple injuries—liver, spleen, and small bowel—and asked how you will proceed. You may be also presented with a penetrating case with right upper quadrant gunshot wound.

How to Answer?

Start with the basic trauma algorithm
  Primary survey with ABCs
  Simultaneous resuscitation
  Secondary survey with head-to-toe physical examination
    when the primary survey is complete and patient is
    stabilized
  C-spine immobilization
  Chest and pelvis x-ray in the trauma bay
  Unstable patient gets FAST or DPL in trauma bay—if
    positive, then operate immediately
  Stable patient is most likely evaluated with a CT scan
Nonoperative Management
  Nonoperative management is for patients with blunt
    trauma, minimal other injuries, no indications for

abdominal exploration, and no hemodynamic instability. Also, the patient should ideally have normal mental status and no severe traumatic brain injury.
Bedrest in monitored setting (ICU or stepdown), NPO, IVF, serial hemoglobins
Consider angiography and embolization for patients with liver injury identified on CT scan (large injury, IV contrast blush, and/or pseudoaneurysm)
Have a low threshold to take to the OR
Operative Management
  Prep chin to knees
  Midline incision
  Four quadrant packing
  Rapid abdominal survey and control any intestinal spillage
  Mobilize liver (divide falciform, triangular/coronary ligaments)
Always place drains to control bile leak
1. Simple laceration—direct pressure, topical hemostatic agents (i.e., SurgiCel, Avatine), cautery, argon beam coagulator
2. Deep laceration—finger fracture and ligation of individual vessels, liver suture to reapproximate injured area, pack laceration with vascularized tongue of omentum mobilized from transverse colon
3. Extensive injuries (bilobar, hepatic venous injury, retrohepatic cava)—decide early to use "damage control" surgery
   (a) Mobilize liver
   (b) Gauze packing anteriorly and posteriorly to tamponade bleeding
   (c) Temporary abdominal wall closure
   (d) Angioembolization via interventional radiology
   (e) Return to the OR in 12–36 h after resuscitation to correct hypothermia, acidosis, and coagulopathy. Plan to ask for help (trauma surgeon, liver surgeon, transplant surgeon) and have ample blood products available. You can even offer to transfer with open abdomen to a higher level of trauma care at a level 1 trauma center.
4. Hepatic vein injury—Use Pringle maneuver (vascular clamp across the portal triad) to help diagnose. Pringle controls inflow. If major hemorrhage stops, bleeding is from the hepatic artery and/or portal vein. If bleeding does not stop, it is from the hepatic veins or retrohepatic inferior vena cava.
   (a) Consider total hepatic isolation and/or atriocaval (Shrock) shunt. Place Rummel tourniquet around infrahepatic (suprarenal) IVC, perform a median sternotomy, open the pericardium, place a Rummel tourniquet around intrapericardial IVC, then try an atriocaval shunt (chest tube down through hole in right atrium and below level of liver injury)

Postoperative Management

  Consider endoscopic retrograde cholangiopancreatography (ERCP)—especially useful for patient with bile leaking from drains. ERCP and biliary stent can decrease pressure at sphincter of Oddi and help bile outflow preferentially via the CBD and help leak from injured live seal.

  Fever is common—work up for all infectious causes; if no cause is found, then you can attribute to liver injury alone.

Common Curveballs

Patient becomes coagulopathic intraoperatively (switch to packing and "damage control")

Patient has a transfusion reaction

Patient has associated intra/extra abdominal injuries (you can pack abdomen to deal with them)

Patient has retrohepatic caval injury

Patient has postoperative abscess or biloma (percutaneously drain)

No simple methods of controlling bleeding work

Examiner asks you how to perform the Pringle maneuver

Patient develops postoperative hemobilia/hepatic artery pseudoaneurysm (angiographic embolization)

Patient who underwent nonoperative management for a known liver injury becomes septic from small bowel injury

Clean Kills

Performing a CT scan in an unstable patient (do FAST or DPL and if/when positive, take directly to surgery)

Attempting nonoperative management when not indicated (e.g., hemodynamically unstable patient or severe concomitant brain injury)

Not knowing several operative techniques to control bleeding

Not performing "damage control" when indicated

Not ruling out other injuries prior to going to the OR (for example, missing pneumothorax/hemothorax or open book pelvic fracture in the trauma bay)

Summary

Always follow the standard trauma algorithm to avoid missing an injury, and identify and treat life-threatening injuries first and in a timely manner before launching into details of your operative management. Nonoperative management is preferred for the stable patient, but have a low threshold to operate if the patient becomes unstable or has brain injury or other injuries. Be familiar with techniques to mobilize the liver and repair liver injuries (finger fracture, packing, Pringle maneuver, hepatic isolation), and always carefully assess for associated injuries and leave a drain. Remember to use damage control techniques for the cold, coagulopathic, acidotic patient. Also remember that interventional radiology techniques are much advanced currently, and many liver injuries are amenable to angioembolization in the appropriately selected patient.

Pelvic Fracture

Concept

A high frequency of associated injuries give the force needed to fracture the pelvis. Pelvic fracture is often associated with falls and motor vehicle collisions. Fractures are usually classified by the vectors of force that produced the injury:

Anterior–posterior compression

Lateral compression

Vertical shear

Combined vector injury

Way Question May Be Asked?

"A 33-year-old man is brought into the emergency room after falling off of the second story of a building. He is tachycardic and has a systolic blood pressure of 90. What do you want to do?"

  You may get the scenario with the patient after motor vehicle collision, fall, or crushed in an industrial accident. Be systematic in the workup and on guard for the associated ureteral/rectal injuries and the ongoing blood loss requiring angiography.

How to Answer?

In the trauma setting, always perform the ABCs first:

  Airway and cervical spine (C-spine) control (intubate with C-spine control if necessary)

  Breathing and ventilation (if patient needs a chest tube, place before CXR)

  Circulation and IV access

  Disability (neurologic status)

Do not skip secondary survey either, or you will miss some key finding (high-riding prostrate, blood at urethral meatus, blood on rectal examination)

History should be an AMPLE one:
  Allergies
  Medications
  Past medical history
  Last meal
  Events surrounding trauma
Physical Examination
  Head to toe
  Finger/scope in every hole/orifice
  Pelvic and rectal examination
Diagnostic Studies
  CXR
  Pelvis x-ray
  FAST and/or DPL/DPA
  CT scan abdomen/pelvis if stable (include head if there
    are neurologic signs)

Surgical Treatment

1. Resuscitate the patient and treat any associated life-
   threatening injuries:
   (a) Two large-bore peripheral IVs
       2 L crystalloid (20 cc/kg)—can repeat once if no
       response, followed by blood if hemodynami-
       cally unstable
2. FAST/DPL if you suspect intra-abdominal injury in an
   unstable patient (make the incision above the umbilicus to
   avoid entering pelvic hematoma)
   (a) Take patient to the OR only if grossly bloody; other-
       wise, it is unlikely to be enough hemorrhage to be the
       source of the patient's hypotension
   (b) If grossly bloody, position in lithotomy to be able to
       perform rigid sigmoidectomy to evaluate the rectum
3. Blood at urethral meatus
   (a) Urethrogram first—suprapubic cystotomy if positive
       urethrogram
   (b) Cystogram if urethrogram is negative
   (c) If cystogram is positive, is the injury intra- or extra
       peritoneal?
   (d) Intraperitoneal injury gets primary repair in layers
   (e) All bladder injuries get suprapubic cystotomy
4. If rectal injury:
   (a) Diverting sigmoid loop colostomy
   (b) Presacral drains
   (c) Rectal washout
5. If retroperitoneal hematoma:
   (a) Do not explore unless ruptured or expanding
   (b) If you explore, ligate internal iliacs, pack, and go to
       angiogram for embolization if necessary
6. Stabilize all unstable fractures early with external fixator
   in the emergency department or T-POD Pelvic Stability

Device is a non-metal fabric belt for use with open-book
pelvic fracture patients/bedsheet (after DPL if hemodynamically unstable)
7. Angiogram to embolize bleeders, especially if the patient
   is bleeding externally
8. All open pelvic fractures get a diverting sigmoid colostomy

Common Curveballs

Examiner asks you about associated injuries and how to
  manage (ureteral, rectal, spleen, liver, chest, small bowel,
  pancreas)
Pelvic fracture is unstable
Pelvic fracture is "open"
DPL is grossly positive
DPL is only positive by red blood cell count (do not perform
  a laparotomy first)
Pelvic hematoma is expanding/ruptured
Patient has neurologic injury and is hypotensive with grossly
  positive DPL (examiner is testing your priorities: explore
  abdomen first as this is most life-threatening)
Patient develops deep vein thrombosis (DVT)/pulmonary
  embolism (PE) during hospitalization (scenario switch)

Clean Kills

Not knowing how to proceed or proceeding expeditiously in
  an unstable patient
Not performing DPL in an unstable patient
Performing DPL with an incision below the umbilicus
Not identifying associated injuries
Not knowing what to do with a pelvic hematoma

  FAST examinations are slowly replacing the need for
DPLs. An unstable patient with a positive FAST examination
requires emergent operative intervention. An unstable patient
with a negative FAST examination and a confirmed pelvic
fracture needs emergent interventional radiology (IR) intervention. If IR is unavailable, emergent OR intervention for
preperitoneal packing is warranted.

Summary

**Pelvis fractures represent one of the greatest challenges
to a trauma service. It is important to diagnose whether a
patient is hemodynamically unstable from a pelvic fracture verses another source. Various techniques for hemostasis are available, including interventional radiology,
external compression devices, and preperitoneal packing
in the operating room. These techniques vary by the**

resources available in the hospital setting. Pelvic angiography has become an important modality in controlling hemorrhage and is supported by Level I evidence. Angiography can be repeated if necessary and is relatively safe compared to operative intervention.

Rib Fractures

Concept

Rib fractures can result in severe chest wall pain, chest wall hemorrhage, and in worst cases, chest wall instability. Flail chest is considered when three or more ribs are segmentally fractured. Chest wall instability along with the underlying pulmonary contusion is the driving force behind the respiratory insufficiency that develops.

ABCs
Mechanism
High suspicion for underlying thoracic injuries
    Pneumothorax
    Hemothorax
    Cardiac contusion
Simple
    Aggressive pulmonary toilet
    Adequate pain control
Flail chest
    Aggressive pulmonary toilet
    Careful fluid management
    Pain control (± epidural, intercostal blocks)
    Will be underlying lung contusion
    Follow arterial blood gas (ABG)/CXR
    Selective intubation based on associated injuries/respiratory status
    Selective rib fixation

Summary

Chest wall injuries, including rib fractures, frequently involve trauma, especially blunt trauma. Although the spectrum of thoracic injuries is vast and includes isolated or multisystem trauma-related injuries, it is important to understand the impact of these injuries. The majority of thoracic injuries, including rib fractures, can be managed nonoperatively. It is important to adequately treat the patient's pain to prevent worsening respiratory decompensation. Inadequate pain control can result in poor ventilator weaning, increased and retained secretions, increased physiologic stress response, respiratory failure, and pneumonia. The use of narcotic pain medications, along with regional or local anesthetics, along with nonsteroidal anti-inflammatory drugs (NSAIDs), has

shown great benefits. Rib fixation is still controversial and may benefit a small subset of patients.

Penetrating Neck Trauma

Concept

Mortality from penetrating neck trauma is as high as 10 %, with many important structures in close proximity. Systematic evaluation is necessary and should include evaluation of potential injuries to airway, esophagus, and vascular system. Classically, it is broken down into three zones:

I. Clavicles to cricoid cartilage (proximal carotid, subclavian, vertebrals, esophagus, trachea, brachial plexus, spinal cord, thoracic duct, and upper lung)

II. Cricoid to angle of mandible (carotid, vertebral, jugular, larynx, esophagus, trachea, vagus, recurrent laryngeal, spinal cord)

III. Angle of mandible to base of skull (pharynx, distal carotid, vertebrals, parotid, cranial nerves)

Way Question May Be Asked?

"You are called to the ED to evaluate a young male who sustained a stab wound to the left neck. On examination, the wound is anterior to the sternocleidomastoid muscle (SCM) at the level of the thyroid cartilage." Presentation may vary. You may also be given an injury to the carotid artery, jugular vein, trachea, esophagus, or a combination.

How to Answer?

Always start with advanced trauma life support (ATLS) protocol in all trauma scenarios

    A: Airway (If there is any concern for airway compromise, intubate)

    B: Breathing

    C: Circulation (Make sure to ask for vital signs and always state that you will place two large-bore peripheral IV lins)

    D: Disability (Ask for Glasgow Coma Score [GCS])

    E: Exposure (Especially important in a penetrating mechanism—make sure there are no other injuries)

Remember the AMPLE history:

1. A: Allergy/airway
2. M: Medications
3. P: Past medical history
4. L: Last meal
5. E: Event—What happened?

Secondary Survey
1. Hard Signs of vascular (shock, active bleeding, pulsatile or expanding hematoma) or aerodigestive injury (airway compromise, extensive subcutaneous emphysema, stridor, air leak from neck)
2. Soft signs of vascular (stable hematoma, widened mediastinum) or aerodigestive injury (dysphagia, voice change, hemoptysis)

Management

Hard signs of vascular injury or aerodigestive injury mandate immediate surgical exploration (regardless of zone).

Zone 1: In general, the operative approach requires a median sternotomy to access the right subclavian and innominate artery. A trap door incision may be needed to access the left subclavian artery if left of the midclavicular line.

Zone 2: In general, the operative approach for zone II injuries includes a cervical incision (like elective carotid endarterectomy) along the anterior border of the SCM. This allows for exposure of the major vascular structures (carotid, jugluar) as well as the trachea and esophagus. For isolated tracheal injury, a collar incision (like elective thyroidectomy) can be considered.

Zone 3: In general the operative approach to zone III injuries includes a cephalad extension of the unilateral cervical neck incision. Disarticulation of the mandible may be required. In rare cases, a limited craniotomy may be needed. For all these reasons, nonoperative management and interventional radiology embolization is preferred if possible for vascular injury in this location.

Extra Tricks for Hemorrhage Control

Do not blindly clamp vessels in emergency department (may make injury worse)

Use direct pressure (ideally)

Balloon tamponade (use a Foley catheter, stick into wound and blow up balloon)

Soft signs of vascular injury or aerodigestive injury mandate further workup.

If the patient is hemodynamically normal and there are no hard signs, then a diagnostic workup is considered.

1. CT scan of the neck (include head and chest in most cases) with IV contrast is the first step. This study can identify and specifically locate vascular injury. It can also suggest (although not confirm) aerodigestive injury if air is noticed in the soft tissues.

2. Conventional interventional angiography can identify and locate vascular injury and has the added benefit of allowing treatment in selected cases with embolization and/or stent placement.

3. Duplex ultrasound can be used to examine the carotid artery. However, it does not well visualize vertebral arteries and is limited in proximal and distal regions as well.

4. Flexible/rigid bronchoscopy can be used for evaluation of tracheal injury.

5. Flexible/rigid espohagoscopy can be used for evaluation of esophageal injury.

6. Gastrograffin swallow can be used to evaluate for esophageal injury (it is often best to perform both endoscopy and gastrograffin swallow because each has a small miss rate for injury; combining both methods lowers the miss rate).

Common Curveballs

Patient has combined injuries to multiple structures within the neck

Patient has a tension PTX that causes or contributes to hypotension

Patient has associated chest and abdominal injuries (do not miss other injuries)

Patient has tissue loss and circumferential carotid injury

Patient has operative exposures

Patient has thoracic duct injury

Clean Kills

Not securing the airway

Missing a tension PTX

Delaying an operation in a patient with hard signs

Forgetting to evaluate for aerodigestive injury

Not performing angiography or CT angiogram for Zone I and III (in stable patients)

Discussing ultrasound (except to rule out cardiac tamponade with FAST)

Summary

The neck has a high density of vital structures in a relatively small and unprotected anatomic region. Mortality can be high as 10 % with injuries in this area. Always start with the ABCs of trauma. Always remember all possible injuries (vascular, trachea, esophagus). Operate immediately for hard signs. Perform a complete workup for all patients with soft signs or any concern. Airway compromise from laryngotracheal injuries and hemorrhage from injuries to major vessels are the main causes of rapid death. Many injuries are not apparent on initial evaluation and failure to recognize major airway and

vascular injuries can significantly alter morbidity and mortality. Penetrating neck injuries are categorized according to their anatomic location:

Zone I: Clavicles to cricoid cartilage
Zone II: Cricoid to angle of mandible
Zone III: Angle of mandible to base of skull

Pulmonary Embolism

Concept

Concentrate on pulmonary embolism as a life-threatening complication of surgery or trauma. This will be associated with endothelial injury, stasis, and hypercoagulability (Virchow's triad), often in conjunction with femoral or iliac DVT (although not always known before PE). Do not spend too much time on the workup of inherited hypercoagulable disorders; the point is to proceed to appropriate resuscitation, diagnosis, and treatment.

Way Question May Be Asked?

"You are called to the bedside to evaluate a 56-year-old man on postoperative day 5 after urgent sigmoid colectomy for perforated diverticulitis. He is tachycardic with a heart rate of 115, and is saturating 85 % on 2 L nasal cannula oxygen. What do you do?"

The question may offer additional information, such as mental status changes, anxiety, chest pain (pleuritic or otherwise), temporality of desaturation (acute onset), or hypotension. Preponderance of symptoms may be presented as respiratory or cardiac. Your approach should methodically, but efficiently, sort out which underlying mechanism is really predominating.

How to Answer?

Begin resuscitation as you consider the history and physical examination: Supplemental oxygen (placement if not on, or increased method of delivery—change nasal cannula to face mask/non-rebreather), vascular access, IVF, CXR, EKG, ABG, transfer to ICU (if not already there), potential role for rapid response team (especially if you cannot arrive promptly)
History
    Major risk factors:
        Major general surgery
    Previous venous thromboembolism
        Cancer
        Thrombophilia
Orthopedic hip or knee replacement
Major trauma (especially lower extremity/pelvic fracture, spinal cord injury)
Older age (some cut off at age >40 years, others at > 60 years)
Class III/IV heart failure
    Respiratory failure requiring mechanical ventilation
    Acute stroke with paresis (<3 months)
Symptoms
    Sudden cardiac arrest (PE is on differential)
    Anxiety, altered mental status
    Hemoptysis
    Shortness of breath
    Chest pain, crushing or pleuritic
    Palpitations
Physical Examination
    Vital signs (tachycardia, arrhythmia, pulse oximetry, temperature)
    Mental status
Lung sounds, tachypnea, accessory muscle use, diaphoresis
Neck veins

Diagnostic Tests

CXR—Usually normal. Be sure to state that you are using CXR to rule out other treatable causes for respiratory distress on your differential (CHF/pulmonary edema, effusion, or pneumothorax).

EKG—most common finding is sinus tachycardia. look for signs of right heart strain (ST changes, right axis deviation, right bundle branch block); need to rule out MI

ABG—should show hypoxia and often respiratory alkalosis from hyperventilation

White blood cell count—rule out sepsis

International normalized ratio/PTT—will need baseline

D-dimer—always elevated in patients with PE, but also elevated postoperatively in surgery patients; very helpful to rule out PE if normal

CVP—nonspecific

Echocardiogram—can show right heart failure (enlarged right ventricle); may show clot in pulmonary artery

Ventilation/perfusion (V/Q) scan—this nuclear medicine test is rarely used but may be considered in patients who are high risk for empiric anticoagulation, and who cannot have IV contrast agent

Pulmonary angiogram—gold standard of historical interest; very rarely used

CT angiogram—modality of choice if not contraindicated; needs IV contrast

Extremity duplex ultrasound—should be done to evaluate for concomitant DVT, both for treatment considerations and for risk of further PE propagation; normal duplex does not rule out PE

Treatment

Resuscitation—as noted above; should begin concomitant with history and physical examination

Anticoagulation, weight-based (choose from one option below):

1. Heparin bolus: 80 units/kg + 18 units/kg continuous infusion
2. Low molecular weight heparin (e.g., enoxaparin [Lovenox]): 1 mg/kg every 12 h
   Submassive/massive PE

Anticoagulation as above, plus:

1. Thrombolysis therapy
   (a) Pharmacologic (i.e., tPA)—contraindications include intracranial bleed (stroke, trauma, neoplasm), recent or active internal bleeding (peptic ulcer disease [PUD], etc.), recent major surgery
   (b) Mechanical—If suitable interventional radiology facilities available, it may be useful in patients with contraindication to pharmacologic thrombolysis
2. Surgical embolectomy
   Rarely done, but may be necessary in patient with contraindication or failure of thrombolysis, with impending cardiovascular collapse
   Unless you are cardiac surgeon, do not do this yourself
3. Inferior vena caval (IVC) filter
   Should be considered in:
   (a) Patients with recurrent PE despite therapeutic anticoagulation
   (b) Patients who have undergone mechanical thrombolysis or surgical embolectomy
   (c) Patients who cannot be anticoagulated (contraindication)

Common Curveballs

Patient had recent surgery (trauma, abdominal aortic aneurysm repair, colectomy)

Patient had recent GI hemorrhage (PUD, diverticulitis)

Patient has intracranial hemorrhage

Patient has IV contrast allergy so you cannot do CT angiogram (consider other diagnostic testing, or empiric treatment if not contraindicated)

Patient is pregnant (use heparin only, not Coumadin)

Patient has heparin-induced thrombocytopenia after giving heparin

Patient has recurrent PE while therapeutic (use IVC filter)

Patient presents with hemodynamic instability (impending cardiovascular collapse) with no interventional radiology capabilities (consider medical thrombolysis, surgical embolectomy)

Clean Kills

Delaying resuscitation while spending too much time on history and physical examination, particularly on workup of inherited disorders

Not moving the patient expeditiously to the ICU

Missing a key different diagnosis (sepsis, pneumothorax, MI, cardiac tamponade)

Obtaining radiologic studies (i.e., CT scan) other than CXR prior to starting anticoagulation

Giving thrombolytics to a patient who is freshly postoperative or has other contraindications

Not knowing the indications for IVC filter placement

Summary

PE must remain high on the differential for any patient with new-onset cardiopulmonary symptoms. Rapid simultaneous resuscitation and workup is key to successfully treating the patient. Anti-coagulation is the primary treatment, although more aggressive therapy should be considered in patients with massive or submassive PE.

Splenic Trauma

Concept

The spleen is the most commonly injured organ in abdominal trauma. Splenic injury will occur be in the setting of penetrating or blunt trauma. Gunshot wounds to the abdomen need exploration. Stab wounds can be managed by local wound exploration plus DPL. Blunt trauma requires a CT scan in stable patients and DPL in unstable patients.

Way Question May Be Asked?

"A 60-year-old man is brought into the emergency department after a motor vehicle crash. He was the belted driver and his vehicle was hit on the driver's side. Heart rate is 120 and blood pressure is 120/80. CXR demonstrates left-sided lower rib fractures. How do you proceed from here?"

Scenario may change to a teenager with abdominal trauma, a patient who is initially hemodynamically unstable, or a patient with a concomitant intracranial injury. You may also already be in the OR for another cause and find a splenic injury intraoperatively.

How to Answer?

Always start with ATLS protocol in all trauma scenarios:
  A: Airway
  B: Breathing
  C: Circulation (Make sure to ask for vital signs and always state that you will place two large-bore peripheral IVs)
  D: Disability (Get GCS; management may change if have head injury)
  E: Exposure (Especially important in a penetrating mechanism—do not miss other gunshot wounds)
Remember the AMPLE history
Include secondary survey—look for associated injury in blunt trauma (e.g., pelvic/extremity fracture)
Diagnostic Testing
    Laboratory panels (make sure to always include type and cross match)
    CXR/pelvis x-ray, spine workup (if blunt trauma)
    FAST ultrasound
    If hemodynamically unstable and positive, proceed to the OR for exploratory laparotomy
    If hemodynamically stable, then obtain a CT scan if reasonable (even if FAST positive):
    CT scan (usually pan CT—head, cervical spine, chest, abdomen, pelvis) with IV contrast
Resuscitate
    Always place two large-bore peripheral IVs
    Administer 2 L of *warm* crystalloid
    Consider early blood product (packed red blood cells [PRBCs] and fresh frozen plasma [FFP])

Surgical Treatment

Perform an exploratory laparotomy in any patient who is hemodynamically unstable, regardless of age. Most of these patients get a splenectomy.
For a penetrating mechanism, you need to rule out left-sided diaphragmatic injury and other associated injuries (heart, liver, stomach, pancreas, kidney, colon, small bowel, etc.)
In the OR:
  (a) Make a generous midline incision (mention that you will not go below the umbilicus if you suspect pelvic fractures with pelvic hematoma)
  (b) Pack all four quadrants, determine the source of bleeding (know how to describe placement of a supraceliac aortic clamp)
  (c) Perform splenorrhaphy only if hemodynamically normal, no brain injury, younger patient, lower-grade injury, and there is no other major abdominal injury (i.e. liver). Always consider/mention in pediatric patients. Common techniques include argon beam coagulation, topical sealants, pledgeted repairs, mesh wrapping, and partial splenectomy.
  (d) For splenectomy, mobilize the spleen, ligate short gastrics, and ligate and divide vessels in hilum. Ideally the ligate splenic artery and vein separately to prevent arteriovenous fistula. Be careful to avoid pancreatic injury. Leave a drain for concern of pancreatic tail injury.
  (e) Do not perform autotransplantation.
  (f) Do not forget to vaccinate the patient (prior to discharge if performing splenectomy). This prevents overwhelming postsplenectomy sepsis (OPSS) due to *Streptococcus pneumoniae*, *Haemophilus influenzae*, and *Neisseria meningitidis*.
Nonoperative Management
  (a) In blunt trauma, the patient must be hemodynamically stable.
  (b) A low-grade injury (grade 1–3) has a higher likelihood of success. You are more likely to fail with a higher grade.
  (c) Patient should be <55 years of age. Patients older than 55 years have a high nonoperative failure rate.
  (d) There should be no associated intracranial injury because head injury patients will not tolerate hypotension (need to prevent secondary brain injury).
  (e) You can consider interventional radiology (IR) if the patient is hemodynamically normal and has arterial blush seen on CT scan or higher grade injury (typically IR is unavailable on the oral boards).

Common Curveballs

Patient has other associated injuries (head injuries are common)
Patient initially qualifies for nonoperative management but will then fail (usually presents with acute tachycardia and drop in hemoglobin—immediate surgery/splenectomy)
Patient undergoes splenorrhaphy but then develops hemorrhagic shock postoperatively (immediate reoperation and splenectomy)
Patient develops OPSS (did you forget vaccines?)
Patient has postoperative pancreatic leak (did you forget to mention possible pancreatic tail injury and drain?)
Patient develops splenic bed abscess (consider drainage, try not to operate)
Patient becomes septic on the floor (missed small bowel injury during nonoperative management)

Clean Kills

Forgetting the ABCs

Missing another cause of shock/hypotension (i.e., hypertension [HTX]/PTX)

Not placing two large-bore IVs

Wasting time with a CT scan in a hemodynamically unstable patient

Not being able to describe trauma laparotomy

Missing early signs of bleeding during attempted nonoperative management

Performing splenorrhaphy in a patient with a head injury

Performing splenorrhaphy in a patient with severe liver injury undergoing damage control surgery

Performing autotransplantation of the spleen

Forgetting to vaccinate the patient and not understanding OPSS

Summary

Splenic injuries are the most common abdominal injury in blunt trauma patients and are frequently the site of clinically significant injury. Both blunt and penetrating mechanisms can occur. Over the last several years, there is increasing awareness that not all splenic injuries require splenectomy. It is important to keep in mind that splenic injuries can be deadly and that patients with splenic injury can bleed to death.

Damage Control Surgery

Concept

During the last several years, there have been a number of advances in trauma surgery that have significantly decreased morbidity and mortality. One of these has been the recognition that damage control surgery saves lives and has become standard of care in certain cases of severe trauma.

Way the Question May Be Asked?

"A 27-year-old man is brought to the emergency department after sustaining a GSW to the right chest and abdomen. He is tachycardic (pulse 140) and hypotensive (BP 80/50 mm Hg). A chest tube is placed in the right chest and yields 1,600 mL of blood. What do you want to do from here?"

Another possible scenario is blunt abdominal trauma in a patient with similar vital signs and positive FAST examination.

How to Answer?

Start with the ABCs of trauma/ATLS while you make sure to have plan for immediate surgery:

A: Often patients are combative and agitated from hemorrhagic shock; it is important to consider early control of the airway (intubation).

B: Chest tube placement is critical as it allows decompression of the pleural space and determines therapy.

C: Place two large-bore IVs for volume resuscitation. Consider activation of massive transfusion protocol if available. Early transfusion of blood products (often called "damage control resuscitation") is important. Minimize crystalloid and give blood products instead. Consider 1:1:1 ratio of PRBC:FFP:platelets.

D: GCS may be depressed from shock alone (especially in penetrating trauma).

E: Obtain thorough exposure to look for all injuries. Do not miss other gunshot wounds.

In the OR:

(a) It is a difficult decision of which cavity to explore first. Many cases like this will need both laparotomy and thoracotomy. Plan and prepare for both so you do not have to re-prep and drape. Do not be afraid to switch in the middle.

(b) Start with laparotomy if you are given a GSW to the abdomen and an unstable patient. You may not need thoracotomy even if the initial chest tube output is >1,500 mL. This may be the liver bleeding up through a hole in the diaphragm that stops with diaphragm repair and liver packing.

(c) Damage control principles include wide exposure, control hemorrhage, control GI contamination, and temporary closure of the surgical incision (i.e., VAC closure).

(d) Remember to warm the patient as much as possible in the operating room.

(e) Transport to the ICU for resuscitation.

Patients who are likely to need damage control (early pattern recognition):

1. Penetrating thoracic or abdominal trauma and SBP<90
2. Penetrating abdominal injury in patient with concomitant extremity vascular injury
3. Blunt abdominal trauma and SBP<90 with positive FAST
4. Open book pelvic fracture with abdominal injury
5. Shotgun wound to the femoral triangle of the thigh or a mangled extremity from blunt trauma
6. Thoracotomy or laparotomy that is to be followed by another procedure (i.e., craniotomy, interventional radiology, etc.)
7. Lethal triad (severe acidosis, hypothermia, and coagulopathy)

Intraoperative indications to consider damage control:

Physiologic Reasons

(a) Initial body temperature (temp $< 35°C$)

(b) Initial acid base status (pH < 7.2, lactate > 5, base deficit < -15 in patient < 55 years of age, or base deficit < -6 in patient > 55 years of age)

(c) Coagulopathy (PT or PTT greater than 50 % above baseline)

Anatomic Reasons

(a) Complex injury (i.e., pancreatico-duodenal) that will take a long complex operation to fix in a patient with physiologic derangement

(b) Missing abdominal wall soft tissue (i.e., shotgun wound)

Techniques for temporary abdominal closure

(a) Towel clips or suture closure of the skin (historical—do not perform now)

(b) Temporary silo closure (Bogota bag—sew IV bag to skin edges)

(c) Vacuum-assisted device closure (commercially available product or homemade version with occlusive/adherent dressing)

Common Curveballs

Examiner describes several injuries and asks for management of each individually and in order of importance

Examiner switches to another body region in the middle of the case

Examiner asks you to describe your resuscitation strategy

VAC system not available (you must know other techniques for temporary closure; i.e., Ioban over drains hooked to suction)

Examiner asks you for techniques of definitive closure of incisions

Clean Kills

Not appropriately and promptly resuscitating the patient

Not starting blood products early

Missing tension PTX

Not having full exposure and missing an injury

Failing to recognize that the patient needs damage control

Trying to definitively fix all injuries at the initial operation

Not operating on an exsanguinating patient

Not planning for and prepping both the chest and abdomen before starting surgery and not adding other incisions in a timely fashion

Performing splenorhaphy (rather than splenectomy) in patient getting abdominal damage control

Summary

The overall approach includes abbreviated operative times, delaying definitive repair of injuries, and temporary closure. Transfer to the ICU allows for resolution of the severe acidosis, hypothermia, and coagulopathy (the "lethal triad") before returning to the operation for definitive surgical repair. This is most commonly done for abdominal injury, but can be used in chest, extremity, and neck injuries as well. Formal closure of thoracotomy and laparotomy incisions can prove to be time consuming, leading to worsened outcomes and other complications such as abdominal compartment syndrome.

Thoracic Trauma

Concept

Thoracic trauma is a major cause of mortality. Life-threatening problems should be treated as soon as they are identified. You must identify and treat the following life-threatening conditions promptly:

Tension pneumothorax

Cardiac tamponade

Massive hemothorax

Tracheobronchial tree injuries

Traumatic aortic injury (blunt aortic injury—BAI)

Way Question May Be Asked?

"You are called to the ED to see a 25-year-old man who suffered a GSW to the chest. His HR is 130 and his SBP is 70/palp. What do you want to do?"

The point of the question is to test your ability to manage an unstable patient.

How to Answer?

Start with a plan to do multiple simultaneous things while planning for possible emergency surgery. Take a brief history and perform a physical examination as you start resuscitating the patient/getting ready to transport patient to the OR (IV access, laboratory tests, etc.):

- AlgorithmABCs (airway first!)
- Resuscitation (IVF/blood, full set of labs, NGT, Foley)
- Past medical history, medications, allergies (if possible to obtain this information)
- FAST ultrasound—most important to rule out pericardial effusion (can also see HTX/PTX in experienced hands)
- On CXR, look for the following:
  HTX

PTX

Bullets

Flail chest/rib fractures

Signs of BAI (widened mediastinum, hemothorax, apical cap, depressed left mainstem bronchus, deviated NGT)

Physical Examination

Vital signs (if unstable, address life-threatening issues as you identify them)

Distended neck veins and hypotension (tamponade, tension pneumothorax)

Chest auscultation (to determine pneumothorax, HTX)

Head-to-toe physical examination (do not miss any gunshot wound holes)

Do not remove any foreign bodies (remove in OR)

Subcutaneous emphysema, "sucking chest wound," flail chest

Diagnostic Tests

CT scan (never in an unstable patient!)

Angiogram (any patient with suspicion of traumatic rupture of aorta/BAI—this has mostly been replaced by CT scan, but need to know as backup or "gold standard"

Remember that traumatic aortic rupture does not explain hypotension in a blunt trauma patient—look for another source (abdominal bleeding, pelvic fracture, etc.)

Surgical Management

Know when to place a tube thoracostomy/chest tube!

No breath sounds—Unstable patient: you do not need a CXR; place chest tube before confirming with CXR

Know the indications for ED thoracotomy

Penetrating trauma with cardiac arrest

"Signs of life" in the field and lost en route to ED (maximum 15 min)

Perform through the fifth intercostal space with a left anterolateral incision and rib spreader. Hold lung superiorly with a sponge stick or assistant's hand and in order:

1. Open pericardium anterior to phrenic nerve

2. Clamp descending aorta above diaphragm (feel for NGT to make sure you do not clamp esophagus)

Hope to find and fix cardiac tamponade

More likely to salvage patient with stab than gunshot wound

Do not get suckered into doing ED thoracotomy in blunt trauma

Dead is dead—unless patient loses vitals right in front of you in ED

Know indications for a pericardial window

– Transmediastinal GSW, even if the patient is stable

– Dilated neck veins/high CVP and patient in shock

– Indeterminate FAST

– FAST negative with associated hemothorax (can empty pericardial blood into pleural space)

After chest tube is placed, know when surgery is indicated

1. Initial chest tube output > 1,500 cc (some go with 1 L)

2. Chest tube output >200 cc/h for 4 consecutive hours

Know what to deal with through a throracotomy:

1. Bleeding from chest tube (see numbers above)

2. Large air leak with hypoxemia (check tube and system first to make sure surgery really indicated)

3. Esophageal injury in chest (right thoracotomy unless distal third esophagus)

4. Left subclavian and/or descending aortic injury

Know what to deal with through a median sternotomy:

1. Suspected cardiac injury (positive pericardial window or pericardial FAST)

2. Left supraclavicular stab wound

3. Suspicion of great vessel injury (pulmonary hilum)

4. Suspicion of injury to right inominate artery (cannot reach this through anterolateral thoracotomy)

5. Tracheal injury

6. Allows access to heart, ascending aorta, inominate, proximal right subclavian, right carotid

Diaphragmatic Injuries

Must have a high index of suspicion (no good radiologic test—CT, MRI, ultrasound)

Look for NGT that goes down normally into stomach then comes back up into left chest

In patients with a left-sided throacoabdominal penetrating injury, you need to do laparoscopy to look at the diaphragm. You do not need to do it right because the liver prevents bowel herniation.

There are many ways to repair (one or two layers, pledget or nonpledgeted), but most agree on nonabsorbable sutures.

Consider a gastrostomy tube to hold the stomach in place with a large defect

Repair transabdominally if diagnosed early. If diagnosed late, use a thoracic incision to avoid intrabdominal adhesions.

You may need a mesh if there is a very large defect.Mediastinal InjuriesDo not forget to do a bronchoscopy, esophagoscopy, and gastrograffin swallow to rule out tracheobronchial/esophageal injuries in penetrating trauma.Blunt Cardiac InjuryRarely the cause of shock in trauma patients

Must consider in all patients with blunt chest trauma

Check EKG—if EKG abnormalities are found, then observe on telemetry

Most common arrhythmia is sinus tachycardia

Echocardiography will diagnose contusion, dyskinesia, tamponade, valvular injury

If there are any ischemic changes, treat as an MI patient in ICU

Troponin can be helpful (if normal) to rule out blunt cardiac injury

CPK is less useful because it is elevated from muscle injury-Flail ChestAggressive pulmonary toilet

Careful fluid management

Pain control stepwise increase (NSAIDs, narcotics, epidural, intercostal blocks)

Epidural is the best pain management for broken ribs!

Be aware that the patient will have an underlying lung contusion

Follow ABGs/CXR

Selective intubation based on associated injuries/respiratory status

Common Curveballs

Examiner asks the indications for thoracotomy (blunt vs. penetrating trauma)

Examiner asks when to place chest tube

Examiner asks when to take to OR

Examiner asks when to do angiogram to rule out aortic injury

Patient has widened mediastinum on CXR, hypotensive with distended belly (The problem is in the belly! Always do laparotomy first. Great indication for damapge control.)

Patient has tracheal/esophageal injury (Do not forget to perform bronchoscopy/esophagogastroduodenoscopy)

Patient has visceral herniation through diaphragmatic injury (explore in OR)

Examiner asks about the best exposure for the injury (i.e., limitations of a median sternotomy)

Patient has concomitant traumatic brain injury (which do you approach first?)

Patient has obvious intraabdominal injury (which do you approach first?)

Examiner asks where aortic injury typically occurs and how to repair

Patient has contralateral injury

Patient has postoperative thoracic duct leak or postoperative empyema

Clean Kills

Forgetting about the ABCs

Failing to do an ED thoracotomy when indicated

Failing to place a CT tube when indicated

Asking for CXR to confirm tension PTX

Missing/failing to consider/diagnose blunt aortic injury

Performing a CT scan in an unstable patient

Not knowing how to repair diaphragmatic injury

Summary

Examiners will be interested in determining if you know when and when not to get additional tests versus moving directly to operating room for pericardial window, thoracotomy, or median sternotomy. Do not forget to start with the ABCs and do not forget to rule out other (nonthoracic) injuries.

Vascular

Brandt D. Jones

Abdominal Aortic Aneurysm

Concept

An aneurysm is defined as a greater than 50 % increase from normal vessel diameter. The annual risk of rupture is less than 1 % if the aneurysm is less than 4 cm, up to 50 % if the aneurysm is greater than 8 cm. There is an increased risk of abdominal aortic aneurysm (AAA) in patients with coronary artery disease, politeal or femoral aneurysm, and genetic collagen diseases.

Way a Question May Be Asked?

"A 56-year-old woman is seen in the emergency room (ER) with complaints of back pain and is hypotensive. Physical examination is notable for a pulsatile epigastric mass."

Rarely will the patient present with the classic triad of flank/back/abdominal pain, hypotension, and pulsatile mass above the umbilicus. You should also be prepared for the asymptomatic patient referred from a primary physician with an incidental finding of pulsatile abdominal mass or aneurysm found incidentally on computed tomography (CT).

How to Answer?

For an unstable/ruptured patient, take a focused history and physical examination while resuscitating the patient and preparing them for the operating room (OR).

B.D. Jones, D.O. (✉)
General Surgery, University of Medicine and Dentistry of New Jersey, School of Osteopathic Medicine, Stratford, NJ, USA
e-mail: bjones50@gmail.com

Diagnostic Tests
  Bedside ultrasound (stat)
  CT with intravenous (IV) contrast for operative planning (stat)
  Flat or lateral (abdominal) x-ray can be used
Surgical Treatment
  Permissive hypotension: maintain systolic blood pressure (SBP) of 70–80; higher is associated with loss of initial tamponade
  Type and Cross 6 to 10 Units packed red blood cells, large bore IV (above and below diaphragm), Foley, arterial line
  Send the patient to the OR with fresh frozen plasma, cryoprecipitate, and O-negative blood.
  Prepare the patient from neck to knees.
  Anesthetize the patient after they are prepped and draped.
  Use an aortic occlusion balloon if there is rapid deterioration.
Open Repair
  Proximal Control
    Use a transperitoneal approach to control the supraceliac aorta.
    Retract the left lobe of liver to the right.
    Open the gastrohepaticomentum and enter through the lesser sac.
    Retract the stomach and esophagus to the left.
    The aorta is clamped as it exits the cura of the diaphragm (may need to divide cura)
    Allow the anesthesia to catch up and begin blood transfusions.
    If possible, replace clamp of the infrarenal neck if possible once the patient stabilizes.
  Get distal control of both iliacs.
  Enter the hematoma.
  Open the aneurysm and evaluate.
    You may need to ligate the inferior mesenteric or lumbar arteries if there is significant retrograde bleeding.
  Repair with a tube graft.
    Moderate (3–4 cm) iliac aneurysms can be repaired at a later date.

Do not choose aortobifemoral bypass surgery (longer operation).

Close the peritoneum over the graft.

Prepare to deal with hypothermia, acidosis, coagulopathy, postoperative myocardial infarction (MI), abdominal compartment syndrome, renal failure, loss of pulses in an extremity, and reperfusion injury.

Common Curveballs

Aneurysm is suprarenal

Aneurysm is 4 cm

Examiner asks when you will reimplant inferior mesenteric artery (IMA; you do not need to if there is strong back-bleeding or no backbleeding)

Patient has obstructing or near-obstructing sigmoid colon lesion (key to the answer here is size of AAA vs. how close to obstructing is the colon lesion)

Patient had prior transverse colectomy for cancer (need to reimplant the IMA if stump pressure <70 and check arteriogram preoperatively)

Aneurysm presents in an atypical fashion (embolization to the legs, inflammatory, aortacaval fistula, acute AAA thrombosis with pelvic and lower extremity ischemia)

Patient presents later with graft infection, aortoenteric fistula (axillofemoral bypass first, followed by ligation aorta), or pseudoaneurysm at anastomosis

Examiner asks you to describe your preoperative cardiac assessment (stress thallium)

There is an intraoperative anomaly (horseshoe kidney, retroaortic renal vein, left-sided inferior vena cava [IVC])

Patient is in shock (if examiner asks if you want to get a CT or go straight to the OR, go to the OR and resuscitate en route)

Examiner asks what to do with a patient with dementia, with metastatic cancer, or who is elderly

Patient had prior abdominal surgery (colectomy: reimplant IMA)

Examiner asks about your feelings on stent grafts (results are good so far in symptomatic patients, but always be the conservative surgeon on the board examination)

Patient has a common postoperative problems (likely at least one of the following):

Hypothermia

Acidosis

Coagulopathy

Renal failure—(abdominal compartment syndrome, acute tubular necrosis, atheromatous debris, ureteral injury, hypovolemia—a favorite question is postoperative low urine output after AAA)

Loss of pulses in an extremity

Abdominal compartment syndrome

Ischemic left colon (reimplant IMA if stump pressure < 40)

Postoperative MI

Spinal cord ischemia

Impotence

Clean Kills

Not knowing how to gain control of a rupturing aorta

Not prepping the patient widely enough (include neck and thighs—"chin to knees")

Not ruling out MI or other abdominal processes

Not palpating pulses

Addressing AAA first in patient with positive persantine thallium or cardiac catheter

Not knowing how to manage common postoperative problems (see above)

Trying to perform any endovascular stent graft

Not taking an asymptomatic patient with rapid AAA growth to the OR

Risk of Rupture

5-cm AAA: annual risk ~5 %

7-cm AAA: annual risk ~20 %

Acute Extremity Ischemia

Concept

This acute event is characterized by the six Ps: pain, paresthesias, pulselessness, pallor, paresis, and poikilothermy. The severity of symptoms often correlates with the severity of ischemia, with only 6–8 h before irreversible ischemic changes occur if untreated.

Way Question May Be Asked?

"A 63-year-old man was admitted to the hospital after an inferior wall MI. Five days later, he develops sudden-onset acute left leg pain. On examination, his leg is cool to the touch and pulses are absent below the inguinal ligament."

You need to act quickly to avoid having to do a fasciotomy (although you will likely have to describe the procedure anyway). Checking pulses bilaterally at all levels is critical to determining the level of the likely occlusion and plan your operative management. Remember that a history consistent with an embolus does not necessarily rule out other causes!

How to Answer?

History
 Duration of symptoms
  (6–8 h before irreversible muscle necrosis)
 Risk factors
  Other embolic events (cerebrovascular accident [CVA]/
   transient ischemic attack [TIA]/endocarditis)
  Arrhythmia or valvular heart disease
  Recent MI with mural thrombus
  AAA
  Peripheral vascular disease (PVD)
  Extremity bypass surgery
  Hypercoagulable state (e.g., malignancy)
  Recent trauma or surgery (e.g., orthopedic)
 Muscle pain
 Atherosclerotic disease
Physical Examination
 An acute, cool, white, pulseless leg requires emergent
  intervention
 Examine bilaterally
 Document pulses with Doppler
 Conduct neurologic examination
 Ankle-brachial index
 Be mindful of aneurysms (abdominal/femoral/popliteal)
 Bruits/pulsatile masses
Preoperative Workup
 You may not have much time, but you can do an intraop-
  erative angiography.
 Imaging
  CT angiography (imaging of choice for acute ischemia)
  Arteriography (use brachial puncture if femoral pulses
   are absent)
  Duplex ultrasonography (can be done at bedside)
 Two-dimensional echocardiogram (do not delay treatment)
 Coagulation studies
 Creatine phosphokinase, creatinine, and lactate levels (to
  make sure the patient does not develop rhabdomyolyis
  or renal failure)
Nonoperative Treatment
 All patients are started on heparin with bolus loading
 Supplemental oxygen and IV hydration (you are likely
  using contrast and many patients present dehydrated)
 Pharmacologic Thrombolysis
  Acceptable treatment for all embolic acute events
  Lyses clot in both large and small arteries
 Mechanical Thrombolysis
  Particularly useful in bypass graft occlusions
Operative Management
 The history and physical examination direct treatment.
  If dissection is the cause, you will need endovascular
   stenting or reconstruction.
 There is an increasing need for arterial bypass.

Have on-table angiography available.
Prepare the abdomen and bilateral limbs.
 You may need aortic control or to harvest the saphe-
  nous vein.
Obtain proximal and distal control
Administer heparin bolus before clamping
Completion angiography
Be prepared for fasciotomies
Specific Locations
 Absent Bilateral Femoral Pulses
  Explore bilateral groins for saddle embolus
  Prepare the infraclavicular area for possible extra-ana-
   tomic bypass (axillofemoral bypass)
 Absent Unilateral Femoral Pulse
  Iliac origin (embolism or stent occlusion)
  Unilateral groin exploration
 Absent Popliteal Pulse
  Unilateral groin exploration
  May need to expose popliteal artery for continuing dis-
   tal thrombus
 Pre-Existing Superficial Femoral Artery Disease
  Femoropopliteal bypass is the treatment of choice
Previous bypass
 Prepare to expose both anastamoses
 Likely need to revise distal anastamosis if recent
 Vein graft may need to be replaced
Upper Extremity
 Rarely limb threatening
 Expose brachial artery, generally at level of cubital
 Low threshold for surgical exploration
Continue patients on heparin until therapeutic on vitamin K
 antagonist.

Common Curveballs

Patient had recent bypass surgery
Patient has postoperative compartment syndrome
Patient has postoperative rhabdomyolysis
Patient has postoperative acidosis or hyperkalemia from a
 reperfusion injury
Patient needs amputation for severe injury
Examiner asks you to describe the fasciotomies
Aortic embolus needs an extra-anatomic bypass
Young patient needs evaluation for dissection
Pulses do not return after embolectomy

Clean Kills

Trying to avoid the OR (deteriorating patients get explored,
 not taking a fresh postoperative patient back to the OR)
Prepare to revise or replace the graft

Forgetting to anticoagulate preoperatively, intraoperatively, and postoperatively

Forgetting to check pulses preoperatively

Forgetting to check pulses and completion angiography postoperatively

Carotid Stenosis

Concept

Carotid stenosis is usually described as extracranial cerebrovascular disease. Pay attention to the indications for surgery. Be sure to differentiate carotid disease symptoms from rare "posterior" ischemia originating from the basovertebral system.

Way Question May Be Asked?

"A 53-year-old woman is seen in the ED for TIA, which resolved in the next several hours. She is later referred to your office for evaluation of a left-sided bruit."

How to Answer?

History
  MI or cardiac catheterization
  Hypertension
  Diabetes mellitus
  Hypercholesterolemia
  Peripheral artery disease
  History of TIA/CVA
  Other sources
    MI
    Arrhythmia
    Ataxia, gait disturbances, bilateral lower-extremity weakness
    Basovertebral ischemia
    Intracranial physiology
Physical Examination
  Signs of PVD
  Neurologic examination to localize side
  Bruits, may have bilateral disease
  Blood pressure in both arms (to rule out aortic arch disease)
Testing
  Noninvasive
  Carotid duplex ultrasound (first-line imaging)
  Electrocardiogram (EKG)
  CT or magnetic resonance imaging (MRI) of the head/brain
  Computed tomography angiography (CTA)/magnetic resonance angiography (MRA) of the neck and brain for preoperative planning

Indications for Surgery
  Asymptomatic Patients
    >80 % stenosis
    >60 % with simultaneous coronary artery bypass grafting (CABG)
  Symptomatic Patients
    1 CVA or >1 TIA
    >50 % stenosis
    100 % occlusion, do not operate
Medical Treatment
  Beta blockers
  Blood pressure control (SBP <160)
  Antiplatelet
  Statin or other cholesterol management
  Smoking cessation
  Diabetic control
  Excess weight loss
Stenting Considerations (Based on Comorbidities)
  Life expectancy <5 years
  MI in prior 4 weeks, CABG within 6 months
  Congestive heart failure with ejection fracture <30 %
  Dialysis dependent
  Severe chronic obstructive pulmonary disease with FEV1 <1.0 L
  Anatomically high lesions
  Radiation-induced stenosis
Operative Approach
  Place patient in recumbent position with head turned to opposite side.
  Gently prepare the neck.
  Make an oblique incision along the anterior border of the sternocleidomastoid muscle.
  Divide the fascial vein as it comes across the level of the bifurcation.
  Dissect out the common carotid along the medial border to avoid the vagus nerve.
  Expose the common carotid, internal carotid, and external carotid arteries to areas devoid of hard plaque.
  Determine the need for shunting (awake monitoring, cerebral monitoring, carotid stump pressure).
  Administer a heparin bolus before clamping.
  Clamp in disease-free areas, internal carotid artery first.
  Select a shunt (the safest choice on the oral boards is to shunt all patients and perform under general anesthesia).
  Begin arteriotomy on the common carotid artery in a vertical fashion and extend onto the internal carotid artery.
  Back bleed the shunt to free air/debris.
  Lift the artery away from plaque.
  Check for loose flaps. If necessary, tack with double arm 6-0 prolene with knots on the outside of the vessel.
  Close the vessel with a vein patch or Hemashield patch.
  Flush all vessels before the closing patch.
    Release internal carotid artery to flush debris, then reclamp.

Release external carotid artery first to prevent debris/air from entering internal carotid artery distribution

Drains and heparin are physician dependent.

Common Curveballs

Patient has complete occlusion of the common carotid artery

Patient has a postoperative stroke (get a stat ultrasound—likely a dissection)

Patient has 78 % stenosis and is asymptomatic

Patient has 49 % stenosis and is symptomatic

Patient has an ulcerated plaque

Patient had a recent stroke (check CT; if no stroke is shown, administer heparin and perform carotid endarterectomy [CEA] in 1 week; if positive for stroke, perform CEA in 6 weeks)

Patient has restenosis after CEA

Patient has postoperative MI, neurologic deficit in recovery room, headache, or bradycardia in recovery room

Patient has an acute stroke in your follow-up of an asymptomatic lesion (do not rush to operate: Tissue plasminogen activator if <3 h from onset of symptoms; aspirin, physical therapy, and CEA in 6 weeks if after 3 h from onset of symptoms)

Patient has expanding hematoma in neck postoperatively

Patient has plaque that continues into the base of skull

Patient has no appropriate vein to harvest

Patient has postoperative hypotension/hypertension (nasogastric tube/nitroprusside/cardene, volume and dopamine drip)

Patient has nerve injury

Examiner asks about management of crescendo TIAs (go to OR!)

Patient has three-vessel heart disease and 90 % stenosis (CEA+CABG)

Clean Kills

Not being clear on preoperative indications

Not discerning from basovertebral ischemia

Operating on fresh CVA

Not getting a cardiac workup and CTA/MRA preoperatively

Performing a blind endarterectomy (need to visualize endpoints of plaque)

Not being able to describe the methods to minimize internal carotid artery debris

Chronic Lower Extremity Ischemia

Concept

This peripheral vascular disease in the extremities that may present in several ways. Often, the examiners will be testing indications for surgery and nonoperative management of PVD. It is important to remember that chronic diseases affect all arteries, including the renal and coronaries. Look for lesions at major branching points.

Way a Question May Be Asked?

"A 45-year-old man presents to the office for evaluation of pain in his right calf after walking three blocks. He is a smoker, overweight, and is currently on no medications."

How to Answer?

Be specific in your indications for surgery:
    Resting pain
    Nonhealing ulcer
    Gangrene
    Intermittent claudication that fails to improve with nonoperative therapies or impairs the patient's lifestyle

History should focus on risk factors:
    Smoking
    Diabetes mellitus
    Hypertension
    Overweight
    MI
    CVA/TIA
    Buerger's disease

Physical examination should look for signs of vascular disease:
    Examine patient bilaterally!
    Document pulses (will give indication as to level of disease)
    Neurologic examination
    Hairless skin, changes in nails
    Ankle-brachial index
    Check for abdominal/femoral/cervical bruits
    Remember to perform a preoperative cardiac workup

Nonoperative Therapy
    Risk reduction (smoking cessation, weight reduction, glucose control, blood pressure control)
    Graded exercise program
    Antiplatelet therapy (aspirin, Plavix)
    Statin therapy
    Beta-blocker therapy if hypertensive
    Other medications (Trental, Pletal)

Noninvasive Vascular Laboratory
    Duplex ultrasound bilaterally, including the Iliacs
    ABIs (ankle-brachial index less the 0.40 is considered critical limb ischemia)
    Segmental Pulse volume recording (PVR)

Invasive Testing
    Aortogram with distal run-off
    MRA
    CTA with three-dimensional reconstruction

Interventions

    Interventional therapy is recommended only after all attempts at medical therapy have failed.

    Never take a smoker to the OR!

    Endovascular treatment can be recommended for focal lesions in large-diameter vessels (aorta/iliacs).

    Perform open bypass surgery for distal disease, multiple segments, long lesions, and aortoiliac disease.

Operative Approach

    Proximal and distal control

    Intraoperative heparin before clamping

    Use a vein whenever possible (~70 % 5-year patency)

        In Situ or Reverse greater saphenous vein

            If in situ, you must use a valvulotome and tie off all branches.

            Use a preoperative duplex to evaluate the suitability of the vein.

            For saphenous vein harvesting, start proximally and work distally.

            If short, you can use a composite graft.

    Use heparin-bonded polytetrafluoroethylene if you must use a graft.

    The distal target depends on preoperative arteriography.

    Make a vertical incision to expose the femoral artery (allows extension if the exposed area is not suitable to clamping).

    Make a medial incision to expose the popliteal for above-the-knee bypass.

    Exposure of the peroneal and posterior tibial below the trifurcation often requires detachment of the soleus.

    The anterior tibial should be exposed by a longitudinal incision two fingerbreaths lateral to the anterior tibial border.

    Perform a completion angiogram and documentation of pulses in the OR.

Common Curveballs

Patient has postoperative hemorrhage

Patient has postoperative graft thrombosis or infection

Any stent placed occludes

Angioplasty restenoses

Angioplasty leads to vessel dissection

Patient has postoperative compartment syndrome

Patient develops heparin-induced thrombocytopenia

Clean Kills

Not being clear in the indications for surgery

Not trying nonoperative therapy for intermittent claudication

Not knowing the noninvasive vascular studies

Not taking the patient back for immediate postoperative graft thrombosis

Trying to describe a technique you have not performed

Not being prepared for postoperative complications

Not being able to read an angiogram if it is handed to you

Spending.

Acute Deep Vein Thrombosis

Concept

Acute venous thromboembolism (VTE) has several severe consequences, including pulmonary embolism (PE) and postthrombotic syndrome. The three components of Vischow's triad include venous stasis, endothelial injury, and a hypercoagulable state, which lead not only to treatment considerations but also a starting point in the workup of a patient with acute deep vein thrombosis (DVT).

Way a Question May Be Asked?

"A 72-year-old woman was admitted to the intensive care unit following a diagnosis of severe pneumonia requiring respiratory support. Three days later, it is noted that her left lower extremity is swollen more than the right."

You may receive a history of laboratory tests or lines placed in the groin. Alternatively, a young patient may present to the trauma unit after a fracture or injury to the limb.

How to Answer?

History should focus on risk factors:

    Pregnancy or oral contraceptive use

    Injury within the last 3 months

    Central venous lines, laboratory draws, pacemaker placement

    Sedentary lifestyle or long-distance travel

    Malignancy

    Recent surgery

    Paresis

    Age greater than 80

    History of previous DVT

Physical Examination

    Look for signs of compartment syndrome

        Document pulses

        Evaluate active and passive range of motion

        Look for color or temperature discrepancies

        Calf pain or tenderness with compression (Homan's sign)

Initial Testing
  Contrast venography (former criterion standard, now used for clinical trials primarily)
  Duplex ultrasonography:
    Test of choice
    Incompressibility
    Luminal color filling
  D-Dimer (if negative, there is a decreased complication rate)
  Magnetic resonance venography (MRV):
    Less expensive than contrast venography, more expensive than ultrasound
    More reliable detection of non-flow limiting DVT
    More reliable detection of proximal extent
Prophylaxis
  Low risk (2 %):
    Age less than 40 years with no risk factors
    Minor surgery
    No prophylaxis needed
  Moderate risk (10–20 %):
    Age less than 40 years with risk factors
    Age 40–60 years
    Minor procedures
    Mechanical or pharmacologic prophylaxis
  High risk (20–40 %):
    Minor surgery with age >60 years
    Minor surgery with age 40–60 years and risk factors
    Major surgery
    Mechanical or pharmacologic prophylaxis
  Very high risk (40–80 %)
    Major surgery
    Multiple risk factors
    Mechanical and pharmacologic prophylaxis
Treatment
  Elevation and bed rest may help with symptoms, but has no effect on DVT
  Begin anticoagulation as soon as diagnosis made:
  Unfractionated heparin intravenous
  Subcutaneous low molecular weight heparin
  Conversion to Vitamin K-antagonists (VKA) with goal INR of 2.0–3.0
    Example: Warfarin
  Thrombolysis
  Massive or symptomatic DVT
  Restores venous patency
  Evaluate for need for stent
    May–Thurner Syndrome
      Right common iliac artery compresses the left common iliac vein
  Nonmassive PE
    Similar treatment algorithm to DVT
    Consider IVC filter
  IVC Filter
    Prevents PE not DVT

A second PE would be fatal
Thrombolysis or anticoagulation are contraindicated
Follow-up
  Continue treatment for 6 months for the initial event
  Lifelong therapy for recurrent event while on VKA or if second event would likely be fatal
  Repeat ultrasound
    19 % have proximal extension despite adequate anticoagulation therapy at 6 months

Common Curveballs

Patient had recent major surgery
Patient has platelet count <100
Patient has worsening symptoms
Patient has acute shortness of breath

Clean Kills

Holding or delaying therapy
Starting VKA without heparin bridge (skin necrosis)
Not evaluating the proximal extent of thrombus
Not working up a hypercoagulable state or evaluating for malignancy

Venous Stasis Ulcer

Concept

The spectrum of valvular incompetence and chronic venous outflow obstruction has resultant venous hypertension, edema, cellulitis, and ulcers. Valvular incompetence accounts for 90 % of cases, with DVT accounting for the other 10 %.

Way Question May Be Asked?

"A 49-year-old woman (G4P4) comes to your office complaining of pain and swelling in the lower legs, varicose veins, and a nonhealing ulcer on the medial aspect of her right ankle. What do you want to do?"

You may even be given the increased skin pigmentation and the varicosities.

How to Answer?

History
  Vascular disease
  History of DVT

Clotting disorders
Prior treatments
Professions with long periods of standing
Pregnancy
Physical Examination
Complete vascular examination
Varicosities (size, location, firmness)
Calf tenderness/swelling (DVT)
Edema
Brawny induration/discoloration
Dermatitis
Ulceration (most occur medial)
Brodie-Trendelenburg test (Elevate leg until it is drained of venous blood. Place tourniquet below the knee. Have the patient stand and see if more blood flows into varicosities when the tourniquet is released after they fill from arterial pressure (30 s). This tests superficial reflux.)
Diagnostic Testing
Laboratory panels including prothrombin time/partial thromboplastin time, factor V Leiden, proteins C and S, antithrombin III level
Check ABI (if <0.6, question your diagnosis)
Duplex scanning to determine sites of obstruction and incompetence (deep, superficial, perforators) and evaluate for DVT

Surgical Treatment

1. Conservative treatment with:
   Compression therapy
   Leg elevation/antibiotics
   Weekly application of Unna boots
   Topical agents (platelet-derived growth factor, epidermal growth factor)
   If ulcer heals (it won't!), the patient is fitted for graduated compression stockings (30–40 mmHg).
2. For superficial vein incompetence alone, high ligation and stripping of greater saphenous vein surgery in indicated.
3. For superficial and perforator incompetence, subfascial endoscopic perforator veins is indicated.
4. For deep vein obstruction, perform air plethysmography to delineate anatomy and choose the appropriate surgical procedure.
   (a) For deep venous obstruction from femoral/iliac thrombosis, cross-femoral and/or saphenopopliteal bypass is indicated.
   (b) For deep venous reflux, valvuloplasty is indicated.
5. You may also need a split-thickness skin graft for healing of ulcer.

Common Curveballs

Conservative therapy fails
Examiner tries to get you to perform variceal ablation in a patient with deep vein obstruction/incompetent perforators
Examiner asks you to describe physical examination tests (Trendelenburg test)
Patient has associated vascular disease (scenario switch)
Patient is pregnant
Patient had a recent DVT
Patient has some coagulopathy

Clean Kills

Confusing with arterial ischemic ulcer
Not performing adequate history and physical examination
Not trying conservative therapies
Not performing a duplex scan
Performing variceal ablation in a patient with deep vein obstruction (this is an important collateral in these patients and can cripple venous outflow)

Summary

Vascular disease processes in general reflect the progression of disease processes that affect the entire body, not just the major arteries involved at presentation. The key to addressing any subject on the matter is modification of risk factors and an assessment of the cardiac system. It is likely that any conservative measures will fail for examination purposes, but failing to try these initially would be a mistake. Also, with advancements in endovascular therapy, many processes can be initially addressed with attempted endovascular procedures. On the boards, these will fail, occlude, or be malpositioned, so it is vital to know the appropriate open procedures in the end and postoperative management.

History and physical examination are vital to the vascular assessment. Focus on not only the presenting symptoms but also for any history of DVT, TIA, CVA, or cardiac dysfunction. Duration of symptoms can sometimes lead to assessing for embolic sources or primary cardiac dysfunction that needs to be addressed at the same time or before your intervention. Be sure to document a bilateral neurovascular exam bilaterally when assessing the extremities; this not only will identify the level of the lesion but dictate treatment. Imaging should always begin with the least invasive method. Doppler

ultrasound is the standard modality in vascular disease and should be ordered before any angiograms, CTs, or MRIs. EKGs, blood type and cross match, and creatinine levels should also be assessed in the laboratory.

Emergencies obviously need to be addressed in an appropriate manner, but even these have the need for medical management postoperatively. Almost all vascular disease benefits from an antiplatelet agent such as aspirin. Although venous disease will often require anticoagulation with a vitamin K antagonist, arterial disease does not require these medications. Do not forget to include blood pressure control with a beta-blocker, cholesterol-lowering agents, diet modification, compression stockings, and most importantly smoking cessation. It cannot be stressed enough that bypass surgery for chronic disease in a current smoker is an incorrect answer for the exam. Follow-up studies should be performed at the 3- and 6-onth interval point, then annually, and should be done with the same modality for accurate assessment.

Although the field of endovascular surgery has developed enormously over the past two decades—and indeed it may be the initial therapy of choice for proximal large-vessel disease—for oral examination purposes most of these will fail or the patient will not be a candidate for intervention. If you choose to discuss these modalities, know the contraindications to avoid slipping up and advocating endovascular treatment inappropriately. Knocking off the kidneys for aortic aneurysm repair is not acceptable. If the examiner allows you to go down a minimally invasive route, remember to obtain postoperative neurovascular exams and repeat angiography immediately for any potential complications.

For open procedures, proximal and distal control is always paramount. For emergent and uncontrolled bleeding, an occlusion balloon catheter should be inserted until control can be obtained. Remember that access to the aorta in the abdomen or even chest may be required for control to occur. When preparing to clamp any arterial vessel, the patient should be given heparin (100 units per kg) before clamping is initiated. For carotid or prolonged surgeries, shunts may be used to preserve distal perfusion. Arteriotomies are made longitudinally; if any plaque is discovered, it should be removed and the vessel flushed with heparin to look for intimal flaps. Saphenous vein is always the graft of choice for examination purposes; it should be harvested from either leg if available, with residual length saved for possible vein patches. Barring an available vein, heparin-bonded PTFE should be used with external supporting rings if performing an extra-anatomic bypass. Reversal of heparin is done with protamine at closure, but recall that this is an anticoagulant itself and too much will make a patient bleed. Do not forget the completion angiogram to evaluate both restoration of flow and to demonstrate the absence of a distal clot.

Postoperatively, neurovascular checks bilaterally and blood pressure control are crucial. In general, a systolic blood pressure between 100 and 160 is a good goal and should be maintained through cardene or labetalol drips if necessary. Any deterioration in a patient postoperatively should prompt an immediate return to the OR for re-exploration. Include the possibility of intraoperative angiography in your planning for return. Also, IV hydration will play a role in postoperative management, with stress on the kidneys with IV dye loads and possible, sudden, and drastic changes in blood pressure and volume. Urine output measurements with a Foley catheter generally suffice for the purposes here. Again, do not forget to address a patient's health risk factors and smoking on discharge.

In a final word, vascular surgery is a progressive disease and treatment modalities attempt to minimize risk to the patient based on life expectancy. The underriding themes are all based on hemodynamic forces, flow velocities, and end organ perfusion. When backed into a corner, take a step back for a moment and determine the most effective, least invasive way to diagnose the problem and get blood to the affected segment of the body.

Conclusions: Last Curveballs Considerations

Marc A. Neff

As a final conclusion to the information presented in this book, I offer some last words of advice: dress conservatively, do not appear hesitant, do not quote the textbooks or the literature, take a single dose of Imodium and alcohol the night before, and remember that the stress of the examination will do strange things to you.

This chapter concludes with a list of common curveballs to anticipate. We all see these in real life and know how to manage them. However, when the curveball comes at you on the boards, you may find yourself with a mental block and end up with a "swing and a miss." The examiners are trying to determine if you are a safe surgeon and will always try to put you in the "gray zone." Therefore, thinking about the following curveballs ahead of time may help you to avoid a return trip to the oral boards:

The patient with a bowel obstruction had a recent myocardial infarction (MI)

An incarcerated/strangulated hernia reduces on induction of anesthesia

The trauma patient has a multisystem injury, especially abdominal and neurologic trauma

Consultants are not available

The patient needing laparotomy had prior abdominal surgery

There is a synchronous mass in colon cancer

The obstructing left colon cancer has a cecal perforation

The patient has a cervical leak after a Zenker's diverticulectomy

The patient perforates after an upper/lower endoscopy

A percutaneous drain did not work

The patient is hypotensive/hypoxic in the recovery room

The patient has multiple gunshot wounds

The patient has neurologic findings after a gunshot wound to the abdomen

A chest tube placed for a hemothorax clots off and makes you think that the output has truly decreased

The patient with abdominal aortic aneurysm has a postoperative MI, colonic ischemia, or renal failure

The patient started on heparin develops heparin induced thrombocytopenia (HIT)

The low anterior resection leaks (LAR)

Medical therapy (always) fails

The patient with MI throws a clot to the superior mesenteric artery 6 weeks postoperatively

The patient develops a pseudoaneurysm

The patient develops an enterocutaneous fistula after extensive lysis of adhesions (LOA)

Fine needle aspiration is not definitive (in any solid mass)

The sarcoma involves an artery/nerve

The patient with colon cancer has a colovesical fistula

Dissection in the pelvis for diverticulitis/cancer injures the ureter

The colon cancer involves the ureters

The patient with rectal cancer presents with a large bowel obstruction

The young patient with hypertension has a multiple endocrine neoplasia syndrome

The endoscopic retrograde cholangiopancreatography fails to remove an impacted stone or diagnose malignancy

The patient undergoes an uneventful laparoscopic cholecystectomy and develops postoperative jaundice

The gallstone ileus has more than one stone in the small intestine

The pregnant patient needs surgical intervention

The preoperative lymphoscintigraphy for a sentinel lymph node in melanoma will light up two lymph node basins

Sarcoma locally recurs

Atrial fibrillation complicates any scenario

Gastric MALT-oma does not respond to *Helicobacter pylori* treatment

The patient has continued air leak after a lung resection

M.A. Neff, M.D., F.A.C.S. (✉)
Minimally Invasive, 2201 Chapel Avenue West, Suite 100,
Cherry Hill, NJ 08002, USA
e-mail: mneffyhs@aol.com

M.A. Neff (ed.), *Passing the General Surgery Oral Board Exam*,
DOI 10.1007/978-1-4614-7663-4_17, © Springer Science+Business Media New York 2014

Patient has a postoperative abscess

The patient undergoing exploratory laparotomy/splenectomy/ laparoscopic cholecystectomy has an unanticipated ovarian mass

Mobilizing the left colon injures the spleen

Mobilizing the right colon injures the ureter

The colostomy becomes ischemic postoperatively

The patient has a parathyroid or laryngeal nerve injury after thyroidectomy

Vascular grafts thrombose/get infected

The patient with DVT fails medical therapy or develops phlegmasia

The postoperative trauma patient gets abdominal compartment syndrome

Excisional biopsy for ductal carcinoma in situ has positive margins

Stomach cancer is high on the lesser curve adjacent to the gastroesophageal junction

Patient has a pancreatic leak after a Whipple procedure

Duodenal stump blows out on Bilroth Two (BII)

Pancreatitis gets infected

Pseudocyst erodes into adjacent structures (stomach, colon, splenic vessels)

Results of a percutaneous biopsy are (always) inconclusive

References

Bland K, Copeland III E. The breast: comprehensive management of benign and malignant diseases. 4th ed. Philadelphia, PA: Elsevier; 2009.

Cameron JL. Current surgical therapy. 6th ed. Philadelphia, PA: Mosby; 1998.

Cameron JL, Cameron AW. Current surgical therapy. 7th ed. Philadelphia, PA: Mosby; 2001.

Coran A. Pediatric surgery. 7th ed. Philadelphia, PA: Elsevier; 2012.

Gomella LG, Lefor AT, Mann B. Surgery on call. Roseville, NSW: McGraw-Hill; 2003. ISBN 3.

Hood RM. Techniques in general thoracic surgery. Philadelphia, PA: Saunders; 1985.

Koutlas TC, Reid M. The Mont Reid surgical handbook. 3rd ed. St. Louis, MO: Mosby; 1994.

Mulholland M, Lillemoe K, Doherty G, Simeone D, Upchurch Jr G. Greenfield's surgery: scientific principles and practice. 5th ed. Philadelphia, PA: Lippincott Williams & Wilkins; 2010.

Norton L, Stiegmann G, Eiseman B. Surgical decision making. 4th ed. Philadelphia, PA: W. B. Saunders; 1969.

Practice Management Guidelines. Home - The eastern association for the surgery of trauma. http://www.east.org/resources/treatment-guidelines. n.p., n.d.

Schwartz SI, Shires GT. Principles of surgery. 7th ed. New York: McGraw-Hill; 1999.

Skandalakis LJ, Skandalakis JE, Skandalakis PN. Surgical anatomy and technique: a pocket manual. 3rd ed. New York: Springer; 2009.

Souba WW, Fink MP, Jurkovich GJ, Kaiser LR, Pearce WH, Pemberton JH, et al. ACS surgery: principles and practice. 6th ed. New York, NY: WebMD Professional; 2007.

M.A. Neff (ed.), *Passing the General Surgery Oral Board Exam*,
DOI 10.1007/978-1-4614-7663-4, © Springer Science+Business Media New York 2014

Index

M.A. Neff (ed.), *Passing the General Surgery Oral Board Exam*,
DOI 10.1007/978-1-4614-7663-4, © Springer Science+Business Media New York 2014

CPSIA information can be obtained at www.ICGtesting.com
Printed in the USA
LVOW09s1425260614

391872LV00001B/15/P